Pediatric Psoriasis

Anna Belloni Fortina · Francesca Caroppo

Pediatric Psoriasis

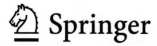 Springer

Anna Belloni Fortina
Pediatric Dermatology Unit, Department of
Medicine DIMED
University of Padova
Padova, Italy

Francesca Caroppo
Pediatric Dermatology Unit, Department of
Medicine DIMED
University of Padova
Padova, Italy

ISBN 978-3-030-90714-3   ISBN 978-3-030-90712-9   (eBook)
https://doi.org/10.1007/978-3-030-90712-9

This Springer imprint is published by the registered company Springer Nature Switzerland AG
The registered company address is: Gewerbestrasse 11, 6330 Cham, Switzerland

Foreword

Psoriasis in children and adolescents is quite often considered rare or infrequent, but one-third of adults with psoriasis report it appeared in their childhood or adolescence.

Psoriasis in children and adolescents is quite often misdiagnosed not only by pediatricians, but also by dermatologists, due to a clinical appearance often different from that typical in adults.

Psoriasis in children and adolescents is often considered a disease affecting only the skin, but it is not rarely associated with comorbidities such as arthritis, obesity, hypertension, metabolic syndrome, and may have an important impact on the quality of life both of the children and of their family.

Finally, some of the treatments used for psoriasis in adults cannot be used or are off-label in children.

Thus, a book on psoriasis in children and adolescents, on its diagnosis and differential diagnosis, comorbidities, quality of life, and therapy is welcome.

Andrea Peserico
Retired Full Professor of Dermatology
and Venereology
University of Padova
Padova, Italy

Preface

"The eye sees what the mind knows"
John W. Budd

We were truly honored when initially asked to consider writing a book dedicated to the specific topic of pediatric psoriasis.

Psoriasis is a chronic inflammatory skin disease with a high prevalence in adults and epidemiological data about childhood psoriasis are constantly increasing worldwide, highlighting an increasing interest about this specific clinical entity among dermatologists and pediatricians.

This book is aimed at dermatologists, pediatricians, medical students, residents, family practitioners, researchers, and nurses, but also to physicians and all other allied pediatric care providers that have an interest in investigating this particular and intriguing clinical entity.

Pediatric psoriasis has several specific clinical characteristics related not only to the clinical manifestations and localization of psoriasis in children, but also to the specific treatments and management in pediatric age.

While building this volume's contents, we have discussed and illustrated several topics related to pediatric psoriasis, supporting our views with the most recent data based on the medical clinical evidence. In each chapter of the book, we described and evaluated several factors involved in the pathogenesis of psoriasis in children, the clinical aspects of the disease, the most recent and proven therapeutic approaches in pediatric age, as well as the widely recognized comorbidities of pediatric psoriasis.

To enhance understanding of the reader, chapters include over 90 original full-color clinical photographs and illustrations, with a special attention and focus on the several clinical types of psoriasis in children. This with the declared aim and the hope to increase awareness of the disease in dermatologists and pediatricians, as dermatology is a medical science principally based on the observation and recognition of skin lesions.

The diagnosis of childhood psoriasis by dermatologists and pediatricians is often more challenging when compared to the well-delineated psoriasis in adults, also considering that formal diagnostic criteria for psoriasis do not exist yet, and that the diagnosis of psoriasis is primarily based on clinical features of skin lesions.

On the other hand, skin biopsy is rarely performed in younger patients, being often reserved for the most difficult or doubtful cases; therefore, a correct diagnosis of psoriasis often depends on the specific experience and on the clinical observation skills possessed by dermatologists and pediatricians. With this guide, our endeavor has been to provide a framework for analyzing clinical signs, developing diagnostic expertise and skills in pediatric psoriasis in pediatricians and dermatologists, all presented in an easily searchable book format.

It has also been our aim to describe specific cardiovascular and metabolic comorbidities which could be associated with psoriasis in children, emphasizing the importance of detecting and managing them, as psoriasis should not be considered a disease involving the skin only; to that purpose, a dedicated chapter is devoted to the impact on quality of life that childhood and adolescent psoriasis has, including the psychological burden in little patients and in family members and caregivers as well.

Psoriasis is a chronic disease, therefore it felt important to highlight and describe the "educational therapy" which should be a well-known tool for dermatologists and pediatricians, as it plays a key role in the multidimensional therapeutic approach that is key in this multifaceted disease.

Educational therapy is indeed crucial for the understanding of the pathophysiology, natural course and consequent management of the disease, not only to the child but also to care providers and family members. In our attempt of being as complete as possible, the review of several topical and systemic therapeutic options actually worldwide available for pediatric psoriasis has been added, that also includes reporting on the increasingly number of available biologic therapies for the treatment of moderate-to-severe psoriasis in children.

In the hope that this work may assist the reader and be a stepping stone for a more thorough understanding of child psoriasis in colleagues, we especially wish to thank all our patients who contribute to give meaning to our daily work, especially in recent global difficult circumstances.

Padova, Italy   Anna Belloni Fortina
Padova, Italy   Francesca Caroppo
December 2021

Acknowledgments

We would like to thank Prof. Andrea Peserico for his wise guidance and support, leading us in the knowledge of the new discoveries and perspectives in the exciting field of pediatric dermatology.

We would also like to thank Dr. Carlotta Bortoletti, Dr. Laura Fagotto, and Dr. Francesca Pampaloni for their contributions to this work.

Contents

1 Introduction.. 1
   1.1 Covid-19 and Psoriasis in Children 4
   References.. 5

2 Epidemiology.. 7
   2.1 Prevalence and Incidence................................... 7
   2.2 Ethnicities and Sex Ratio................................... 9
   2.3 Familiarity 10
   References.. 10

3 Pathogenesis.. 13
   3.1 Genetic Factors 13
   3.2 Environmental Factors....................................... 15
   3.3 Immunopathogenesis... 17
      3.3.1 Skin Cells in Pathogenesis of Psoriasis 17
      3.3.2 Cytokines in the Pathogenesis of Psoriasis 19
   References.. 19

4 Clinical Features 23
   4.1 Clinical Types of Pediatric Psoriasis 26
      4.1.1 Plaque Psoriasis 26
      4.1.2 Scalp Psoriasis 36
      4.1.3 Guttate Psoriasis...................................... 37
      4.1.4 Inverse Psoriasis...................................... 45
      4.1.5 Palmoplantar Psoriasis................................. 50
      4.1.6 Nail Psoriasis 54
      4.1.7 Pustular Psoriasis..................................... 58
      4.1.8 Follicular Psoriasis.................................... 58
      4.1.9 Erythrodermic Psoriasis............................... 62
   References.. 64

5 Diagnosis 67
   5.1 Clinical Severity Assessment................................ 70
      5.1.1 Psoriasis Area Severity Index (PASI).................... 70
      5.1.2 Investigator Global Assessment (IGA) 70

      5.1.3   Physician Global Assessment (PGA).................   72
      5.1.4   Body Surface Area (BSA)   72
      5.1.5   Nail Psoriasis Severity Index (NAPSI),
              Psoriasis Nail Severity Score (PNSS)   72
   5.2   Assessment of Comorbidities   73
      5.2.1   Over-Weight, Obesity, and Central Obesity..............   73
      5.2.2   Hypertension, Hyperlipidemia, and Diabetes Mellitus   74
      5.2.3   Arthritis   74
      5.2.4   Psychiatric Comorbidities   75
      5.2.5   Gastrointestinal Diseases........................   76
   5.3   Assessment of the Quality of Life.........................   76
   References...   77

6 **Differential Diagnosis**   81
   6.1   Guttate Psoriasis.................................   83
   6.2   Inverse Psoriasis.................................   84
   6.3   Plaque-Type and Scalp Psoriasis   84
   6.4   Nail Psoriasis   85
   References...   86

7 **Treatment**...   87
   7.1   Topical Treatments................................   90
      7.1.1   Topical Corticosteroids   91
      7.1.2   Topical Vitamin D Analogues/Vitamin D
              Analogues Combined with Topical Corticosteroids   91
      7.1.3   Topical Calcineurin Inhibitors......................   92
   7.2   Phototherapy   92
   7.3   Systemic Treatments   93
      7.3.1   Retinoids   93
      7.3.2   Cyclosporine   94
      7.3.3   Methotrexate   94
   7.4   Biologic Treatments...............................   95
      7.4.1   Etanercept   95
      7.4.2   Adalimumab.................................   95
      7.4.3   Ustekinumab   96
      7.4.4   Secukinumab   96
      7.4.5   Ixekizumab.................................   97
      7.4.6   Other Biologic Treatments and Small-Molecules Drugs....   97
   7.5   Therapeutic Education and Pro-active Treatment   98
   References...   99

8 **Comorbidities** 101
   8.1   Over-Weight, Obesity and Central Obesity 102
   8.2   Hypertension 103
   8.3   Hyperlipidemia 104
   8.4   Diabetes and Metabolic Syndrome 104

8.5 Psoriatic Arthritis... 106
8.6 Psychiatric Comorbidities 107
8.7 Gastrointestinal Diseases................................. 107
References.. 108

9 **Quality of Life**... 111
9.1 Children's Dermatology Life Quality Index (CDLQI) 112
9.2 Family Dermatology Life Quality Index (FDLQI) 112
References.. 113

Introduction

Psoriasis is a chronic inflammatory immune-mediated skin disease with a prevalence in the global population varying from 2.0% to 8.5%, depending on the study population and other epidemiological factors, such as gender, geographical location, study design, definition of prevalence, and case definition [1–3].

One-third of patients with psoriasis have the onset of disease during childhood and adolescence.

The prevalence of psoriasis in children varies from 0.02% to 0.22% and although the prevalence of the disease is higher in adults than in children, epidemiological data on childhood psoriasis are constantly increasing worldwide [1–3].

Psoriasis results from the interaction among several genetic, environmental, and immunological factors. Patients with psoriasis are genetically predisposed subjects, carrying one or more psoriasis susceptibility genes, in which a dysregulated immune response occurs, following exposure to several trigger environmental factors [2–5].

It has estimated that if one parent of a child is affected by psoriasis, the child has an estimated risk to develop the disease of about 25%, while if the two parents are affected, the child has an estimated risk of 60–70% [6–9].

The increase of prevalence of psoriasis in children in recent years is probably due to the increase of trigger factors in life of people such as physical and mental stress, infections, obesity, and trauma; not less important, the awareness and the attention to physical and skin health are undoubtedly increased in children and adolescents, parents of children, and in physicians in the last decades.

Although psoriasis primarily affects the skin, psoriasis is associated with several comorbidities related to metabolic, cardiovascular, inflammatory diseases and may have a profound long-term impact on quality of life and on psychological health of affected patients.

Data about comorbidities of psoriasis are well-known in adults and more and more evidence are also emerging in children.

A. Belloni Fortina, F. Caroppo, *Pediatric Psoriasis*, https://doi.org/10.1007/978-3-030-90712-9_1

An early recognition of psoriasis and a subsequent adequate approach of the disease in children are essential in order to prevent or to treat considerable comorbidities.

In fact, most of comorbidities in children are related to metabolic disorders (such as over-weight, obesity, central obesity, hypertension, and metabolic syndrome), which could often be treated with simple lifestyle changes (such as eating and physical activities habits), and avoiding drugs, especially if these disorders are recognized in initial phases [9–11].

An early recognition and treatment of psoriasis in children is also important to improve quality of life of affected children, to achieve a psychological comfort and to prevent the appearance of psychological and psychiatric comorbidities, such as anxiety and depression.

Impact on the quality of life could be also related to familial history of psoriasis, as in children with one or both parents with psoriasis, the apprehension of parents could negatively influence the quality of life of the child, also independently of the severity of disease [12, 13].

The diagnosis of psoriasis in children is essentially based on clinical data, so in the process of diagnosis the specific clinical experience, the knowledge, and the ability to recognize clinical signs and the principal clinical characteristics of psoriasis by physicians are crucial.

As in adults, also in children the most common clinical type of psoriasis is plaque psoriasis, which is characterized by sharply demarcated plaques with erythema, silvery, and thickening scales [5–11].

However, children should not be considered "small adults," so childhood psoriasis has specific characteristics related to peculiar morphology of the clinical manifestations, to the localization of disease and also to the specific management and to the possibilities of treatments in pediatric age [13–17] (Fig. 1.1).

About localization of psoriatic lesions, an involvement of the face, scalp, hands, flexural, and anogenital regions is most common in children than in adults and the typical thickened, scaly, erythematous, and well-demarcated plaques, that are generally easy to recognize in adults, are often absent in children.

The most common involvement of areas which are often exposed and visible (such as face, scalp, and hands) may have a strong negative impact on the quality of life of patients, especially in pediatric age, strongly influencing family and social relationships.

Therefore, a correct and complete understanding of all aspects of the disease by physicians in this delicate phase of life of the patient is of great importance.

About treatment of childhood psoriasis, evidence and data are constantly increasing. Many studies investigated the efficacy and safety of several standard psoriasis treatments in children with psoriasis, including topical therapies, systemic therapies, and phototherapy [18–23].

In recent years, the use of biologic treatments in pediatric psoriasis has considerably progressed, showing good results of efficacy and safety of several targeting treatments.

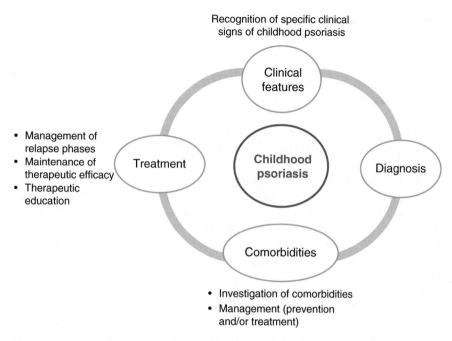

Recognition of specific clinical
signs of childhood psoriasis

Clinical
features

Childhood
psoriasis

Diagnosis

• Management of
  relapse phases
• Maintenance of
  therapeutic efficacy
• Therapeutic
  education

Treatment

Comorbidities

• Investigation of comorbidities
• Management (prevention
  and/or treatment)

Fig. 1.1 Pediatric psoriasis: a multidimensional approach

The objectives of management and treatment in children with psoriasis should be multidimensional and strictly interconnected with the phases of clinical relapse and remission of the disease [18–23].

The treatment of psoriasis in children should be focused on an efficacy management of the clinical relapses, on a maintenance of therapeutic efficacy, and on a prevention of flare-ups [18–23].

In phases of relapse, the treatment of psoriasis is essentially based on the application of topical treatments (such as topical corticosteroids and vitamin D derivatives), but the treatment could also include phototherapy or systemic treatments (such as conventional or biological therapies), according to the severity of the disease and to the impact on the quality of life of child.

A long-term complete remission of psoriasis in children is often difficult to achieve, especially in moderate-to-severe disease, making necessary the use of long-term therapy options [18–23].

Besides the specific treatment of psoriasis in children, not less important is to practice an "educational therapy" addressed by the dermatologists or pediatricians to the parents and family of the child, in order to explain the pathophysiology, the natural course, and the consequent management of the disease [12, 18, 24].

In fact, especially in children with familial history of psoriasis, parents of child are often worried and anxious about the progression of disease.

It should be explained to the parents and to the child that the course of disease is chronic-relapsing, and that the progression is unpredictable, occurring through phases of relapse (often apparently without specific causes) and that the phases of clinical remission can occur after treatment or spontaneously [12, 18, 24].

1.1   Covid-19 and Psoriasis in Children

In December 2019, the severe acute respiratory syndrome coronavirus 2 (SARS-CoV-2) speedily began spreading around the world, resulting in the Coronavirus disease-19 (Covid-19) pandemic.

Few data are available about the impact of Covid-19 pandemic in both adults and children with psoriasis. However, the Covid-19 pandemic and the resulting preventive health measures have certainly greatly influenced in several ways the life of children with psoriasis: in fact, flare-up phases of psoriasis are often related to infection, physical and mental stress, with a high risk of discontinuation of therapies and high risk of psoriasis' worsening during lockdown also due to the difficulties in medical follow-up [25, 26].

About the difficulties in accessing hospitals during lockdown period, some studies have shown that providing an easier access to consultations or teleconsultations could reduce the number of patients discontinuing their therapy. Therefore, this aspect should be improved in order to guarantee an easier access to remote consultations in the management of psoriasis in children with psoriasis [26–28].

The impact of Covid-19 pandemic on patients with psoriasis should be considered as being multidimensional, especially in pediatric age: several patients' associations report that children with psoriasis felt feelings of stigma inside their home and with their family during lockdown periods, showing that the impact of the Covid-19 pandemic and of the confinement measures are far beyond the SARS-CoV-2 infection [27, 28].

Furthermore, lockdown periods forced children and adolescents to stay at home for several weeks and months, away from school and their friends, spending most hours of the day in front of PC and tablets, drastically reducing physical activities and often inducing to eat more and unhealthy food.

Several studies showed that these sedentary behaviors during Covid-19-related lockdown periods have a great negative impact on well-being, mental, physical, and metabolic health of children [27–29].

It is known that children with psoriasis are at high risk of developing other systemic diseases, such as cardiovascular, metabolic, and psychiatric comorbidities. Covid-19 pandemic, confinement measures during lockdown period and related negative changes in lifestyle habits could have further increased the risk of some diseases in children with psoriasis (such as over-weight, obesity, central obesity, hypertension, metabolic syndrome, but also depression and anxiety) [28, 29].

About the treatment and management of psoriasis during the Covid-19 pandemic, there are no specific guidelines and recommendations in pediatric age. However, National Psoriasis Foundation recommends that patients under systemic and biologic treatments for psoriasis should continue their therapies, as evidence does not seem to show that systemic treatments of psoriasis, including immunosuppressive drugs, could significantly impact on the risk of Covid-19 [30].

References

1. Megna M, Napolitano M, Balato A, Scalvenzi M, Cirillo T, Gallo L, Ayala F, Balato N. Psoriasis in children: a review. Curr Pediatr Rev. 2015;11(1):10–26.
2. Relvas M, Torres T. Pediatric psoriasis. Am J Clin Dermatol. 2017;18(6):797–811.
3. Mahé E. Childhood psoriasis. Eur J Dermatol. 2016;26(6):537–48.
4. Forward E, Lee G, Fischer G. Shades of grey: what is paediatric psoriasiform dermatitis and what does it have in common with childhood psoriasis? Clin Exp Dermatol. 2021;46(1):65–73.
5. Eichenfield LF, Paller AS, Tom WL, Sugarman J, Hebert AA, Friedlander SF, et al. Pediatric psoriasis: evolving perspectives. Pediatr Dermatol. 2018;35(2):170–81.
6. Seyhan M, Coskun BK, Saglam H, et al. Psoriasis in childhood and adolescence: evaluation of demographic and clinical features. Pediatr Int. 2006;48:525–30.
7. Eickstaedt JB, Killpack L, Tung J, et al. Psoriasis and psoriasiform eruptions in pediatric patients with inflammatory bowel disease treated with anti–tumor necrosis factor alpha agents. Pediatr Dermatol. 2017;34:253–60.
8. Paller AS, Singh R, Cloutier M, et al. Prevalence of psoriasis in children and adolescents in the United States: a claims-based analysis. J Drugs Dermatol. 2018;17(2):187–94.
9. Mercy K, Kwasny M, Cordoro KM, et al. Clinical manifestations of pediatric psoriasis: results of a multicenter study in the United States. Pediatr Dermatol. 2013;30:424–8.
10. Parisi R, Symmons DP, Griffiths CE, Ashcroft DM. Identification and Management of Psoriasis and Associated ComorbidiTy (IMPACT) project team. Global epidemiology of psoriasis: a systematic review of incidence and prevalence. J Invest Dermatol. 2013;133(2):377–85.
11. Silverberg NB. Update on pediatric psoriasis, part 1: clinical features and demographics. Cutis. 2010;86(3):118–24.
12. Lavaud J, Mahé E. Proactive treatment in childhood psoriasis. Ann Dermatol Venereol. 2020;147(1):29–35.
13. Mercy K, Kwasny M, Cordoro KM, et al. Clinical manifestations of pediatric psoriasis: results of a multicenter study in the United States. Pediatr Dermatol. 2013;30(4):424–8.
14. Tollefson MM. Diagnosis and management of psoriasis in children. Pediatr Clin N Am. 2014;61(2):261–77.
15. Bronckers IM, Paller AS, van Geel MJ, van de Kerkhof PC, Seyger MM. Psoriasis in children and adolescents: diagnosis. Management and comorbidities. Paediatr Drugs. 2015;17(5):373–84.
16. Morris A, Rogers M, Fischer G, Williams K. Childhood psoriasis: a clinical review of 1262 cases. Pediatr Dermatol. 2001;18:188–98.
17. Pinson R, Sotoodian B, Fiorillo L. Psoriasis in children. Psoriasis (Auckl). 2016;6:121–9.
18. Cordoro KM. Management of childhood psoriasis. Adv Dermatol. 2008;28:125–69.
19. Benoit S, Hamm H. Childhood psoriasis. Clin Dermatol. 2007;25(6):555–62.
20. Griffiths CE, Barker JN. Pathogenesis and clinical features of psoriasis. Lancet. 2007;370(9583):263–71.
21. Shah KN. Diagnosis and treatment of pediatric psoriasis: current and future. Am J Clin Dermatol. 2013;14(3):195–213.
22. Dhar S, Banerjee R, Agrawal N, Chatterjee S, Malakar R. Psoriasis in children: an insight. Indian J Dermatol. 2011;56(3):262–5.
23. Mahé E, Maccari F, Ruer-Mulard M, et al. Fédération française de formation continue et d'évaluation en dermatologie-vénéréologie et le GEM Resopso. Psoriasis de l'enfant vu en milieu libéral: les aspects cliniques et épidémiologiques diffèrent des données habituellement publiées. Ann Dermatol Venereol. 2019;146(5):354–62.

24. Randa H, Todberg T, Skov L, Larsen LS, Zachariae R. Health-related quality of life in children and adolescents with psoriasis: a systematic review and meta-analysis. Acta Derm Venereol. 2017;97(5):555–63.
25. Beytout Q, Pepiot J, Maruani A, et al. Association France psoriasis; research group on psoriasis of the French Society of Dermatology (GrPso); research Group of the French Society of Pediatric dermatology (SFPD). Impact of the COVID-19 pandemic on children with psoriasis. Ann Dermatol Venereol. 2021;148(2):106–11.
26. Munster VJ, Koopmans M, van Doremalen N, van Riel D, de Wit E. A novel coronavirus emerging in China – key questions for impact assessment. N Engl J Med. 2020;382(8):692–4.
27. Wosik J, Fudim M, Cameron B, et al. Telehealth transformation: COVID-19 and the rise of virtual care. J Am Med Inform Assoc. 2020;27(6):957–62.
28. Skayem C, Cassius C, Ben Kahla M, et al. Teledermatology for COVID-19 cutaneous lesions: substitute or supplement? J Eur Acad Dermatol Venereol. 2020;34(10):e532–3.
29. Chambonniere C, Lambert C, Fearnbach N, et al. Effect of the COVID-19 lockdown on physical activity and sedentary behaviors in French children and adolescents: new results from the ONAPS national survey. Eur J Integr Med. 2021;43:101308.
30. Gelfand JM, Armstrong AW, Bell S, et al. National Psoriasis Foundation COVID-19 task force guidance for management of psoriatic disease during the pandemic: version 2-advances in psoriatic disease management, COVID-19 vaccines, and COVID-19 treatments. J Am Acad Dermatol. 2021;84(5):1254–68.

Epidemiology

2

2.1 Prevalence and Incidence

In recent years, epidemiological data about the prevalence and incidence of psoriasis are increased, including data about childhood psoriasis.

In fact, in the last decades better data quality resources are available, thanks to ever increasing information collected in large electronic health databases, which are more and more widespread worldwide [1, 2].

The prevalence of psoriasis in the global population ranges from 2.0% to 8.5%, depending on the study population and other several factors which seem to contribute to the prevalence of the disease (such as sex, age, geographical location, genetic and environmental factors, study design, definition of prevalence) [2–4] (Table 2.1).

Several studies report that the incidence of psoriasis shows a bimodal age distribution: a type 1 psoriasis (or "early-onset" or "childhood psoriasis") with an age onset of the disease under 40 years and a type 2 psoriasis (or "late onset" or "adult psoriasis") with an onset after the age of 40 years [2–4].

In type 1 psoriasis, the highest incidence rates are reported between the ages of 16 and 22 years and the median age of onset of childhood-onset psoriasis is between 7 and 10 years of age.

In type 2 psoriasis, the highest incidence rates are reported between 57 and 60 years of age.

However, other studies do not support the existence of these peaks in the age of onset of psoriasis, finding that the incidence of psoriasis increases progressively with the age of the patient up to the seventh decade of life, with a more rapid increase in incidence rate until the age of 30–35 years [3–6].

In about one-third of overall patients with psoriasis, the onset of the disease is reported in pediatric age.

In 10% of children with psoriasis, the disease begins before 10 years of age and in 2% of children before 2 years of age [2–6].

A. Belloni Fortina, F. Caroppo, *Pediatric Psoriasis*, https://doi.org/10.1007/978-3-030-90712-9_2

Table 2.1 Principal data reported in epidemiological studies on childhood psoriasis

Study, period, country	Number of children	Sex distribution (%M; %F)	Age distribution (mean ± SD)	Ethnicity	Family history
Stefanaki et al. 2011, Greece [26]	125	59;41	Range: (1–13) y.o.	81% Greeke	16%
Wu et al. 2011, USA [27]	1361	45;55	(11.8 ± 4.4) y.o. (M) (12.5 ± 4.4) y.o. (F)	n.s.	n.s.
Tollefson et al. 2010, USA [28]	357	48;52	Range: (6.8–14.4) y.o.	n.s.	n.s.
Fan et al. 2007, Cina [29]	277	47;53	Range: 9 months to 15 y.o.	Chinese	8%
Seyhan et al. 2006, Turkey [30]	61	38;62	10.0 ± 4.1	Turkish	23%
Kumar et al. 2004, India [31]	419	52;48	(8.1 ± 2.1) y.o. (M) (9.3 ± 2.3) y.o. (F)	Indian	4.5%
Morris et al. 2001, Australia [32]	1262	47;53	n.s.	n.s.	71%
Raychaudhuri et al. 2000, USA [33]	223	44;56	n.s.	n.s.	68%

M males, *F* females, *SD* standard deviation, *n.s.* not specified, *y.o.* years old

The age at onset of psoriasis is also reported varying with psoriasis clinical subtype; for example, an early disease onset has been reported for pustular psoriasis.

These data could be underestimated, as in adults with psoriasis, although the signs and symptoms of the disease were started in childhood, they might not have been recognized and correctly diagnosed as psoriasis.

In Europe and North America, psoriasis represents 4.1% of all dermatoses observed in pediatric population, but this data is probably underestimated as some patients with mild psoriasis may not come to the physician's attention or may be misdiagnosed [1–3].

Furthermore, in contrast to Europe and North America, childhood psoriasis seems to be almost absent in some epidemiological studies on pediatric dermatoses in Asia, suggesting that psoriasis results from a complex interaction between environmental factors in genetically predisposed patients.

About the prevalence of psoriasis in children, the lowest value is reported in Asia (0.02%), while in Australasia and in Western Europe the prevalence is about 0.21–0.22% [1, 2, 6–9].

The prevalence of disease in children and adolescents under 20 years seems to increase more rapidly in girls compared with boys, suggesting a possible interaction between sex and the development of the psoriasis phenotype in children.

The reported overall age- and sex-adjusted annual incidence of pediatric psoriasis is 40.8 per 100.000 person years [9, 10].

The incidence of psoriasis in children increases with age, varying from 13.5 per 100.000 person years (under 3 years of age) to 53.1 per 100.000 person years (14–18 years of age) [9–11].

The incidence of psoriasis in pediatric population is reported strongly increasing in recent years, becoming more than double in the last 30 years; this data is probably due to the increase of exacerbating factors in life of people such as physical and mental stress, infections, obesity, and trauma [10–14].

Other increasing trigger factors which should be considered in the etiopathogenesis of childhood psoriasis include the use of certain drugs such as lithium, β-adrenergic antagonists, and tumor necrosis factor alpha (TNF-α) inhibitors which are currently used in children with chronic inflammatory diseases, such as juvenile idiopathic arthritis or Crohn's disease [5, 10–16].

Not less important, the awareness and the attention to physical and skin health are undoubtedly increased by young patients, parents of children, and physicians in the last decades.

2.2   Ethnicities and Sex Ratio

Comparing children of different ethnicities, the prevalence of psoriasis is highest in Caucasian children, who also report an earlier mean age of onset, probably due to genetic factors.

Furthermore, the incidence of psoriasis is reported associated with latitude, increasing with the distance from equator [13–17].

About sex, several studies show that the prevalence and incidence of psoriasis in children are higher in girls than in boys and in girls the onset of the disease appears to be earlier (Table 2.2).

Table 2.2 Epidemiological data about pediatric psoriasis

Prevalence	0.02% (East Asia) – 0.21/0.22% (Australasia/Western Europe)
Incidence	13.5–53.1/100.000 person years
Age at onset	• 10% of children: Onset of psoriasis before 10 years of age; • 2% of children: Onset of psoriasis before 2 years of age
Ethnicities	Caucasian children are the most affected, also reporting an earlier mean age of onset
Sex ratio	• Higher prevalence of childhood psoriasis in girls than in boys; • Earlier onset of psoriasis in girls than in boys; • Higher prevalence of scalp psoriasis and lower prevalence of nails involvement in girls than in boys
Familiarity	• 30% of children with psoriasis have familial history of psoriasis with at least one affected first-degree relative; • A child with one parent affected by psoriasis has an estimated risk to develop disease of 25%; • A child with the two parents affected by psoriasis, the child has an estimated risk to develop disease of 60–70%

Compared to male, female children also show some differences regarding the clinical aspect of psoriasis with a higher prevalence of scalp psoriasis and a lower prevalence of nails involvement [14–17].

2.3   Familiarity

Patients with psoriasis are genetically predisposed subjects, carrying one or more psoriasis susceptibility genes, in which a dysregulated immune response occurs, following exposure to several trigger environmental factors (such as mental and physical stress, trauma, infections, drugs, etc.) [5, 14–21].

Although the specific genetic determinants still remain unclear, several family studies support the existence of a genetic predisposition to psoriasis, showing higher incidence of psoriasis in patients with family history of psoriasis, compared with the general population [1, 5, 15–22].

Genetic predisposition to psoriasis results as a complex genetic trait, resulting from genetic and epigenetic factors, related to gene–gene and gene–environment complex interactions.

The prevalence of psoriasis in first-degree and second-degree relatives seems higher in type 1 (child-onset) psoriasis, in comparison to type 2 (adult-onset) psoriasis [17–25].

Approximately 30% of children with psoriasis have a familial history of psoriasis with at least one affected first-degree relative, but the association between a family history of psoriasis and an early disease onset of the disease remains still uncertain. Furthermore, familial history of psoriasis seems to be more related to the paternal branch (Table 2.2).

If one parent is affected by psoriasis, the child has an estimated risk to develop the disease of about 25%, while if the two parents are affected, the child has an estimated risk to develop psoriasis of 60–70% [1, 5, 16, 21, 22].

References

1. Mahé E. Childhood psoriasis. Eur J Dermatol. 2016;26(6):537–48.
2. Parisi R, Symmons DP, Griffiths CE, et al. Identification and Management of Psoriasis and Associated ComorbidiTy (IMPACT) project team. Global epidemiology of psoriasis: a systematic review of incidence and prevalence Global epidemiology of psoriasis: a systematic review of incidence and prevalence. J Invest Dermatol. 2013;133:377–85.
3. Gelfand JM, Weinstein R, Porter SB, et al. Prevalence and treatment of psoriasis in the United Kingdom: a population-based study. Arch Dermatol. 2005;141:1537–41.
4. Augustin M, Glaeske G, Radtke MA, et al. Epidemiology and comorbidity of psoriasis in children. Br J Dermatol. 2010;162:633–6.
5. Eichenfield LF, Paller AS, Tom WL, et al. Pediatric psoriasis: evolving perspectives. Pediatr Dermatol. 2018;35(2):170–81.
6. Burden-Teh E, Thomas KS, Ratib S, et al. The epidemiology of childhood psoriasis: a scoping review. Br J Dermatol. 2016;174:1242–57.
7. Yamamah GA, Emam HM, Abdelhamid MF, et al. Epidemiologic study of dermatologic disorders among children in South Sinai, Egypt. Int J Dermatol. 2012;5:1180–5.

8. Chang YT, Chen TJ, Liu PC, et al. Epidemiological study of psoriasis in the national health insurance database in Taiwan. Acta Derm Venereol. 2009;89:262–6.
9. Bonigen J, Phan A, Hadj-Rabia S, et al. Impact de l'âge et du sexe sur les aspects cliniques et épidémiologiques du psoriasis de l'enfant. Données d'une étude transversale, multicentrique francˌaise. Ann Dermatol Venereol. 2016;143:354–63.
10. Mercy K, Kwasny M, Cordoro KM, et al. Clinical manifestations of pediatric psoriasis: results of a multicenter study in the United States. Pediatr Dermatol. 2013;30:424–8.
11. Al-Mutairi N, Manchanda Y, Nour-Eldin O. Nail changes in childhood psoriasis: a study from Kuwait. Pediatr Dermatol. 2007;24:7–10.
12. Huerta C, Rivero E, Rodriguez G. Incidence and risk factors for psoriasis in the general population. Arch Dermatol. 2007;143:1559–65.
13. Alexis AF, Blackcloud P. Prosiasis in skin of color: epidemiology, genetics, clinical presentation, and treatment nuances. J Clin Aesthet Dermatol. 2014;7:16–24.
14. Ozden MG, Tekin NS, Gurer MA, et al. Environmental risk factors in pediatric psoriasis: a multicenter case-control study. Pediatr Dermatol. 2011;28:306–12.
15. Paller AS, Singh R, Cloutier M, et al. Prevalence of psoriasis in children and adolescents in the United States: a claims-based analysis. J Drugs Dermatol. 2018;17(2):187–94.
16. Relvas M, Torres T. Pediatric psoriasis. Am J Clin Dermatol. 2017 Dec;18(6):797–811.
17. Parisi R, Iskandar IYK, Kontopantelis E, Augustin M, Griffiths CEM, Ashcroft DM. Global Psoriasis Atlas. National, regional, and worldwide epidemiology of psoriasis: systematic analysis and modelling study. BMJ. 2020 May;28(369):m1590.
18. de Jager ME, de Jong EM, Meeuwis KA, et al. No evidence found that childhood onset of psoriasis influences disease severity, future body mass index of type of treatments used. J Eur Acad Dermatol Venereol. 2010;24:1333–9.
19. Odinets A. The incidence of skin diseases in Stavropol territory in 2010–2016. Klinicheskaya Dermatologiya i Venerologiya. 2017;16(6):32.
20. Jacob C, Meier F, Neidhardt K, et al. Epidemiology and costs of psoriasis in Germany a retrospective claims data analysis. Value Health. 2016;19:A566.
21. Megna M, Napolitano M, Balato A, et al. Psoriasis in children: a review. Curr Pediatr Rev. 2015;11(1):10–26.
22. Silverberg NB. Update on pediatric psoriasis. Cutis. 2015;95(3):147–52.
23. Springate DA, Parisi R, Kontopantelis E, Reeves D, Griffiths CEM, Ashcroft DM. Incidence, prevalence and mortality of patients with psoriasis: a U.K. population-based cohort study. Br J Dermatol. 2017;176:650–8.
24. Vena GA, Altomare G, Ayala F, et al. Incidence of psoriasis and association with comorbidities in Italy: a 5-year observational study from a national primary care database. Eur J Dermatol. 2010;20:593–8.
25. Di Meglio P, Villanova F, Nestle FO. Psoriasis. Cold Spring Harb Perspect Med. 2014;4(8):a015354.
26. Stefanaki C, Lagogianni E, Kontochristopoulos G, et al. Psoriasis in children: a retrospective analysis. J Eur Acad Dermatol Venereol. 2011;25(4):417–21.
27. Wu JJ, Black MH, Smith N, et al. Low prevalence of psoriasis among children and adolescents in a large multiethnic cohort in southern California. J Am Acad Dermatol. 2011;65(5):957–64.
28. Tollefson MM, Crowson CS, McEvoy MT, et al. Incidence of psoriasis in children: a population-based study. J Am Acad Dermatol. 2010;62:979–87.
29. Fan X, Xiao FL, Yang S, et al. Childhood psoriasis: a study of 277 patients from China. J Eur Acad Dermatol Venereol. 2007;21:762–5.
30. Seyhan M, Coskun BK, Saglam H, et al. Psoriasis in childhood and adolescence: evaluation of demographic and clinical features. Pediatr Int. 2006;48:525–30.
31. Kumar B, Jain R, Sandhu K, et al. Epidemiology of childhood psoriasis: a study of 419 patients from northern India. Int J Dermatol. 2004;43:654–8.
32. Morris A, Rogers M, Fischer G, et al. Childhood psoriasis: a clinical review of 1262 cases. Pediatr Dermatol. 2001;18:188–98.
33. Raychaudhuri SP, Gross J. A comparative study of pediatric onset psoriasis with adult onset psoriasis. Pediatr Dermatol. 2000;17:174–8.

Pathogenesis

3

Psoriasis is a complex multifactorial disease, histologically characterized by a hyperproliferation of the keratinocytes and an increased rate of turnover-cells in the epidermis.

The pathogenesis of psoriasis involves multiple mechanisms with a complex interaction between genetic, immunological, and environmental factors (Table 3.1).

In the last decade, the advancement of research and knowledge allowed a substantial progress in the understanding of the mechanisms involved in the pathogenesis of psoriasis.

3.1   Genetic Factors

Genetic factors play a key role in the etiopathogenesis of psoriasis. The most important risk factor for psoriasis is the family history of psoriasis, especially in children.

If one parent is affected by psoriasis, the child has an estimated risk to develop the disease of about 25%, while if the two parents are affected, the child has an estimated risk to develop psoriasis of 60–70% [1].

Several studies report that the incidence of psoriasis shows a bimodal age distribution: a type 1 psoriasis (or "early-onset" or "childhood psoriasis") with an age onset of the disease under 40 years and a type 2 psoriasis (or "late onset" or "adult psoriasis") with an onset after the age of 40 years. In type 1 psoriasis, the highest incidence rates are reported between the ages of 16 and 22 years and the median age of onset of childhood-onset psoriasis is between 7 and 10 years of age.

In type 2 psoriasis the highest incidence rates are reported between 57 and 60 years of age.

Type I seems to be an inherited disease, associated with HLA (particularly HLA-C:06:02), while type II is a sporadic disease, not associated with HLA. The prevalence of psoriasis in first-degree and second-degree relatives seems higher in type 1 (child-onset) psoriasis than in type 2 (adult-onset) psoriasis [2, 3].

Table 3.1 Most common environmental factors which can act as trigger factors of psoriasis

Physical skin trauma ("*Koebner phenomenon*")	• Allergic and irritant contact dermatitis • Scratching • Removal of adhesive bandages • Insect bites • Burns • Radiation • Cuts, abrasions • Tattoos
Infections	• Streptococcus pyogenes infections • Staphylococcus aureus infections
Drugs	• Lithium • Antimalarials • Interferon-α • TNF-α inhibitors • β-blockers • Nonsteroidal anti-inflammatory drugs • Tetracyclines • ACE-inhibitors • Terbinafine
Over-weight and obesity	• Higher prevalence of over-weight/obesity in psoriatic patients compared to the general population • Obese patients have higher risk of developing more severe forms of psoriasis
Hormonal factors	• A high percentage of psoriasis seems to begin in puberty • Psoriasis seems to be aggravated by estrogen therapy
Habit of alcohol and smoking	• Higher prevalence of smokers in patients with psoriasis than in the general population, especially in women • Higher risk of developing psoriasis and having a more serious illness in smokers than in non-smokers
Physical and mental stress	• Many patients report the exacerbations of psoriasis associated with a mental or physical stress • In children and adolescents, mental stress could be due to several events (such as separation of parents, family conflicts, school-related stress, difficult social relationships, bullying episodes, etc.)

Genetic predisposition to psoriasis results as a complex genetic trait, resulting from genetic and epigenetic factors, related to gene–gene and gene–environment complex interactions.

Ten chromosomal loci associated with psoriasis susceptibility (PSORS1-PSORS10) have been identified. PSORS1 seems to be the region associated with the greatest risk of psoriasis and it is responsible for approximately 35–50% of the heritability of the disease [4, 5].

PSORS1 resides in the locus gene of Major Histocompatibility Complex (MHC) located on chromosome 6. Although the identification of the causative gene in this locus is very difficult, HLA-C seems to be the causative gene and normal HLA-Cw6 allele seems to be the susceptibility allele in PSORS1 region [4, 6–9].

In psoriatic lesions, CD8+ T cells are mostly found in the epidermis, while CD4+ T cells are predominantly in the dermis. Antigens are presented by HLA-Cw6 to CD8+ T cells, which are MHC class I limited [10, 11].

Psoriasis may be related not only to HLA-Cw6 but also to other MHC class I risk variants [9]. Clonal expansion of CD8+ T cells in the epidermis may occur when HLA-Cw6 presents one or more specific antigens to CD8+ T cells [12].

Genes associated with psoriasis have been noted to be involved in several biological pathways such as antigen presentation, T (Th17) cell differentiation, NF-κB-mediated signaling, IFN signaling, IL-23-IL-17 signaling, alterations of the epidermal barrier, the function of dendritic cells and macrophages, and the responses of keratinocytes [13].

IL-23 signaling stimulates the survival and proliferation of Th-17 cells, which produce IL-17, IL-22, and TNF-α and play a key role in the defense of epithelia from extracellular pathogens [14]. IL-23 signaling also seems to be particularly involved in the pathogenesis of childhood psoriasis.

The response of keratinocytes seems to be an association between psoriasis and the expression of genes during the epidermal differentiation which are located with the epidermal differentiation complex. PSORS4 maps to chromosome 1q21 and includes the epidermal differentiation complex (EDC) [15, 16]. Deletion of the late cornified envelope genes LCE3B and LCE3C, which are contained in the EDC complex, is strongly associated with psoriasis [17, 18]. These 2 genes encode proteins involved in the terminal differentiation of keratinocytes and are overexpressed in psoriasis, wound healing, and following skin injury [19].

3.2   Environmental Factors

Environmental factors play an important role in the pathogenesis of psoriasis, involving physical skin trauma, infections, drugs, over-weight and obesity, hormonal factors, habit of alcohol and smoking, physical and mental stress. Some of these trigger factors could be very relevant in the onset of psoriasis in children and adolescents.

Mechanical skin trauma can trigger a flare-up of psoriasis or the development of new lesions; this phenomenon is known as the "Koebner phenomenon." Factors that may induce Koebner's phenomenon include acupuncture, vaccinations, scratching, removal of adhesive bandages, insect bites, burns (thermal, chemical, surgical), radiation, incisions, cuts, abrasions, tattoos, allergic, and irritant contact dermatitis and phototoxic dermatitis [20]. Koebner phenomenon may be due to the alteration of the epidermal barrier related to trauma and the subsequent events occurring in the dermis. In fact, after a trauma there is an activation of the innate immunity and a subsequent activation of specific immunity, epidermal hyperplasia with hyperproliferation of keratinocytes, and development of angiogenesis [21].

Another possible trigger factor involved in the onset or in the clinical flare-up of psoriasis, especially in pediatric age, is related to infections.

Psoriasis could be associated with Streptococcus pyogenes infections, especially the clinical type of guttate psoriasis and in pediatric age [22]. Guttate psoriasis is more frequently triggered by pharyngeal infections, but also occurs following Streptococcus pyogenes skin infections. The possible role of antibiotics or tonsillectomy in the treatment of guttate psoriasis is still debated and several studies show conflicting data [23]. Superantigens such as Streptococcus pyogenes exotoxin and peptidoglycan can lead to the development of psoriasis due to the altered response of innate immunity to the superantigens. Other microorganisms that may trigger or exacerbate psoriasis are Staphylococcus aureus, Candida, H. Pylori, and Malassezia [24].

It has been shown that many drugs can be responsible for the onset or exacerbation of psoriasis, both in adults and in children. The drugs that may cause psoriasis exacerbation are lithium, antimalarials, interferon-α, TNF-α inhibitors, beta-blockers, nonsteroidal anti-inflammatory drugs, tetracyclines, imiquimod, ACE-inhibitors, terbinafine, and gemfibrozil (fibrates) [25–27]. The mechanisms underlying drug-related psoriasis still need to be fully clarified. Certain drugs may induce hyperproliferation of keratinocytes and interact with the IL-23/IL-17 axis.

Lithium is supposed to cause the exacerbation of psoriasis by interfering with the release of calcium within the keratinocytes through depletion of inositol. Low intracellular calcium levels lead to an increase in proliferation and lack of differentiation of keratinocytes [24].

As for beta-blockers, they are thought to interfere with intracellular cAMP levels: cAMP is an intracellular messenger that promotes cell differentiation and inhibition of proliferation; in fact, beta-blockers work by reducing intraepidermal cAMP levels, and therefore induce hyperproliferation of keratinocytes [28]. The mechanism by which imiquimod causes drug-related psoriasis involves an action on plasmacytoid dendritic cells (pDCs) and a stimulation of IFN-α production, which amplifies both innate and Th1 immune responses [29].

In the suspicion of drug-related psoriasis it is necessary to stop the suspected drug, replacing it with an alternative medication.

Particular attention must be paid to corticosteroids: in fact, although psoriasis may be responsive to treatment with oral corticosteroids, the risks are both tachyphylaxis and the rebound effect.

The most frequent effects of abrupt discontinuation of oral corticosteroids are the rebound phenomenon of the disease and the development of unstable psoriasis.

Among environmental factors, several studies show that alcohol consumption is increased in patients with psoriasis compared to the general population and may even worsen psoriasis, both in adults and in adolescents [30].

Although the link between alcohol and the pathogenesis and exacerbation of psoriasis still remains to be clarified, there is a positive correlation between alcohol abuse and the severity of psoriasis, with a reduced efficacy of treatment and an increase in the mortality rate [31, 32].

About cigarette smoking, the percentage of smokers is higher in patients with psoriasis than in general population, especially in women [33, 34]; the risk of developing psoriasis, having a more serious illness and developing psoriatic arthritis seems higher in smokers than in non-smokers [35, 36]. Smoking may stimulate the onset and persistence of psoriasis due to several immunological mechanisms [30]. The intensity of cigarette smoking (number of cigarettes/day) and duration of smoking seem to be also associated with the severity of psoriasis [37, 38].

Another possible environmental factor is related to over-weight and obesity. Among psoriatic patients, both in adults and in children, there is an increased prevalence of obesity compared to the general population and obese patients are more likely to have severe forms of psoriasis [33, 35, 39–41]. Adipose tissue secretes several pro-inflammatory adipokines such as TNF-α, IL-6, leptin, and adiponectin, which induce a state of low-grade inflammation in patients. This inflammatory state contributes to the pathogenesis of psoriasis [42–44].

Physical and mental stress represent other important environmental factors which could be involved in the onset or flare-ups of psoriasis, especially in children and adolescents. A high percentage of psoriatic patients (from 37% to 88%) associate the exacerbations of psoriasis to a mental or physical stress [45]. Mental stress could be due to several events in the life of children (such as separation of parents, family conflicts, school-related stress, difficult social relationships, bullying episodes, etc.).

The link between stress and pathogenesis of psoriasis is not yet well clarified, but it seems related to the modulation of the hypothalamic–pituitary–adrenal axis, inducing a reduction in cortisol levels due to the stressful factors that could trigger psoriasis exacerbations [46].

Some hormonal factors (e.g., elevated estrogen levels) may also play a role in triggering psoriasis, especially in adolescents. This hypothesis is supported by the finding of cases of psoriasis arising in puberty, cyclic psoriasis related to the menstrual cycle, and psoriasis aggravated by estrogen therapy [47].

3.3 Immunopathogenesis

3.3.1 Skin Cells in Pathogenesis of Psoriasis

Alterations in the innate and adaptive skin immune responses are responsible for the development and maintaining of psoriatic inflammation [48, 49].

An activation of the innate immune system driven by endogenous danger signals and cytokines characteristically coexists with an autoinflammatory perpetuation in some patients, and T cell-driven autoimmune reactions in others [50].

External insults (such as trauma, infections, drugs, and other factors already discussed) can damage keratinocytes, inducing them to release cationic antimicrobial peptides (AMPs)— cationic proteins and members of the innate immune system that contribute in the protection against pathogens, and self-nucleotides, particularly in genetically predisposed patients. The most importance AMPs are cathelicidin (LL-37), defensins, and S100 proteins. Altered keratinocytes also produce chemokines such as CC-chemokine ligand 20 (CCL20) that attract myeloid dendritic cells (mDCs) and TH-17 [48, 51]. The keratinocytes are the major source of AMPs which are synthesized in the stratus granulosum, packaged into lamellar bodies, and then released into the stratus corneum. In skin, AMPs link the innate and adaptive immunity via chemotaxis of dendritic cells and T cells and maturation and activation of dendritic cells [48, 50].

Self-nucleotides can form complexes with antimicrobial peptides which are released from damaged keratinocytes, which can bind to the receptors expressed by antigen-presenting cells (dendritic cells—DCs). These interactions induce a clonal expansion of antigen-specific CD8+ T lymphocytes. This process may occur in the dermis (activation of memory T cells) or in the locoregional lymph nodes (activation of naive T cells). Therefore, activated CD8+ T lymphocytes migrate to the epidermis, where they interact with MHC type I receptors on the surface of keratinocytes (and possibly also melanocytes) and trigger the local release of soluble factors (such as cytokines, chemokines, and mediators of innate immunity), which finally increase inflammation and stimulate keratinocyte proliferation [50, 52–54].

The complex relationship between the various cell types found in the skin, including macrophages, dendritic cells, T lymphocytes, and other immunity cells, is closely dependent on cytokines and chemokines that regulate the complex pathogenesis of psoriasis. Differentiation of Th1 and Th17 cells is stimulated by dendritic cells through IL-23. Adaptive and innate immunity cells (macrophages, mast cells, granulocytes) produce lots of mediators that induce and maintain the characteristics of psoriatic skin at the dermal (e.g., endothelial cells) and epidermal (keratinocytes) levels [55–58].

Endothelial cells express the receptor for VEGF, which induces the proliferation and expression of adhesion molecules at the endothelial level in order to recruit other inflammatory cells. These factors stimulate neo-angiogenesis and lead to the characteristic tortuous appearance of the dermal vessels in psoriatic skin, which contributes to the Auspitz sign [52].

In addition to inflammation and hyperproliferation, neo-angiogenesis is the third key point in pathogenesis. The impaired function of endothelial cells is related to the inflammatory cascade and to the production of several pro-angiogenic factors. Endothelial cells also show an increased expression of adhesion molecules which facilitate the recruitment of circulating leukocytes into the skin [55].

Langerhans cells also play a relevant role in the pathogenesis of psoriasis. Langerhans cells produce TNF-α and IL-23, which induce an increased polarization of naive T cells into Th-17 cells and subsequent IL-17 production. This pathogenic pathway appears to be the most significant in chronic plaque psoriasis [56, 59].

Antigen presentation and a complex network of pro-inflammatory and adhesion molecules optimize T-lymphocyte activation and dermal release of IL-12 and IL-23 by DC cells, promoting Th-1 and Th-17 responses.

Natural killer (NK) cells are also implicated in the early stages of the innate response due to their cytotoxic activity and the rapidity with which they produce cytokines including IFN-γ, which promotes the Th-1 response, and IL-4, which promotes the development of Th-2 [53].

Moreover CD8+ T lymphocytes are greatly increased in psoriatic skin and are also a source of key cytokines in pathogenesis, including IL-17A, TNF, and IL-22 [52].

Recently a new group of cells, involved in psoriasis's pathogenesis, has been described: innate lymphoid cells (ILC). These cells produce IL-17 and IL-22 and express IL-23R, thus representing a direct target of IL-23, inducing IL-17 and IL-22 production [49, 50].

3.3.2 Cytokines in the Pathogenesis of Psoriasis

TNF-α is a pro-inflammatory cytokine produced by several cells, including macrophages, lymphocytes, keratinocytes, Langerhans cells, and endothelial cells. TNF-α induces secondary mediators (IL1, IL6, IL8, NF-kB), adhesion molecules (selectins, cell adhesion molecule 1) which facilitate circulating cells recruitment, and VEGF that stimulates neovascularization [50, 60]. In particular, TNF-α increases production of IL-23 by mDC and, along with IL-17, increases keratinocytes hyperproliferation. TNF-α also increases the production of IL-12 and IL-18 that induce the production of IFNγ and consequently IL-8.

IL-6 stimulates the differentiation of T-naive into Th-17 via signal transducer and activator of transcription 3 (STAT3) pathway [61–64]. STAT3 is a transcription factor that is activated by several cytokines and growth factors, such as IL-6, IL-23, interferons, and epidermal growth factor (EGF). In T-naïve cells, IL-6 stimulates the phosphorylation of STAT3 by JAK and the translocation to the cell nucleus. STAT3 thus activates several genes involved in the differentiation, activation, proliferation, and survival of the cells and also promotes the expression of IL-23R [65]. IL-23R is necessary to confer Th17 full effector functions through the interaction with IL-23 and maintains the amplification and proliferation of Th-17 cells [66].

Th17 effectors stimulate the proliferation of keratinocytes, reduce their differentiation with subsequent parakeratosis, and overall promote an inflammatory response [50]. Among the numerous pro-inflammatory cytokines produced, chemokines attract T lymphocytes and neutrophils, and cytokines of IL1 family, particularly IL36, stimulate the further production of IL6, IL23, IL8, and IL17.

In different clinical subtype of psoriasis, the expression and predominance of involved cytokines differ [58]. In fact, while plaque psoriasis is dominated by TNFα-IL23-IL17 axis, in pustular psoriasis the cytokines principally involved are IL-1β, IL-36α, and IL36γ. Moreover, children affected by psoriasis have a significantly higher levels of IL-22, IL-23 and significantly lower levels of IL-17 than adults [67].

References

1. Swanbeck G, Inerot A, Martinsson T, Wahlström J. A population genetic study of psoriasis. Br J Dermatol. 1994;131(1):32–9.
2. Gudjonsson JE, Kárason A, Antonsdóttir AA, et al. HLA-Cw6-positive and HLA-Cw6-negative patients with psoriasis vulgaris have distinct clinical features. J Invest Dermatol. 2002;118(2):362–5.
3. Henseler T, Christophers E. Psoriasis of early and late onset: characterization of two types of psoriasis vulgaris. J Am Acad Dermatol. 1985;13(3):450–6.
4. Mahil SK, Capon F, Barker JN. Genetics of psoriasis. Dermatol Clin. 2015;33(1):1–11.
5. Capon F. The genetic basis of psoriasis. Int J Mol Sci. 2017;18(12):2526.
6. Veal CD, Capon F, Allen MH, et al. Family-based analysis using a dense single-nucleotide polymorphism-based map defines genetic variation at PSORS1, the major psoriasis-susceptibility locus. Am J Hum Genet. 2002;71(3):554–64.
7. Nair RP, Stuart PE, Nistor I, et al. Sequence and haplotype analysis supports HLA-C as the psoriasis susceptibility 1 gene. Am J Hum Genet. 2006;78(5):827–51.

8. Capon F, Munro M, Barker J, Trembath R. Searching for the major histocompatibility complex psoriasis susceptibility gene. J Invest Dermatol. 2002;118(5):745–51.
9. Okada Y, Han B, Tsoi LC, et al. Fine mapping major histocompatibility complex associations in psoriasis and its clinical subtypes. Am J Hum Genet. 2014;95(2):162–72.
10. Paukkonen K, Naukkarinen A, Horsmanheimo M. The development of manifest psoriatic lesions is linked with the invasion of CD8 + T cells and CD11c + macrophages into the epidermis. Arch Dermatol Res. 1992;284(7):375–9.
11. Bos JD, Hagenaars C, Das PK, Krieg SR, Voorn WJ, Kapsenberg ML. Predominance of "memory" T cells (CD4+, CDw29+) over "naive" T cells (CD4+, CD45R+) in both normal and diseased human skin. Arch Dermatol Res. 1989;281(1):24–30.
12. Chen L, Tsai TF. HLa-Cw6 and psoriasis. Br J Dermatolog. 2018;178(4):854–62.
13. Tsoi LC, Stuart PE, Tian C, et al. Large scale meta-analysis characterizes genetic architecture for common psoriasis associated variants. Nat Commun. 2017;8:15382.
14. Bettelli E, Oukka M, Kuchroo VK. T(H)-17 cells in the circle of immunity and autoimmunity. Nat Immunol. 2007;8(4):345–50.
15. Mischke D, Korge BP, Marenholz I, Volz A, Ziegler A. Genes encoding structural proteins of epidermal cornification and S100 calcium-binding proteins form a gene complex ("epidermal differentiation complex") on human chromosome 1q21. J Invest Dermatol. 1996;106(5):989–92.
16. Capon F, Novelli G, Semprini S, et al. Searching for psoriasis susceptibility genes in Italy: genome scan and evidence for a new locus on chromosome 1. J Investig Dermatol. 1999;112(1):32–5.
17. de Cid R, Riveira-Munoz E, Zeeuwen PL, et al. Deletion of the late cornified envelope LCE3B and LCE3C genes as a susceptibility factor for psoriasis. Nat Genet. 2009;41(2):211–5.
18. Zhang XJ, Huang W, Yang S, et al. Psoriasis genome-wide association study identifies susceptibility variants within LCE gene cluster at 1q21. Nat Genet. 2009;41(2):205–10.
19. Niehues H, van Vlijmen-Willems IM, Bergboer JG, et al. Late cornified envelope (LCE) proteins: distinct expression patterns of LCE2 and LCE3 members suggest nonredundant roles in human epidermis and other epithelia. Br J Dermatol. 2016;174(4):795–802.
20. Weiss G, Shemer A, Trau H. The Koebner phenomenon: review of the literature. J Eur Acad Dermatol Venereol. 2002;16(3):241–8.
21. Ji YZ, Liu SR. Koebner phenomenon leading to the formation of new psoriatic lesions: evidences and mechanisms. Biosci Rep. 2019;39(12):BSR20193266.
22. Norrlind R. The significance of infections in the origination of psoriasis. Acta Rheumatol Scand. 1955;1(2):135–44.
23. Owen CM, Chalmers RJG, O'Sullivan T, Griffiths CE. A systematic review of antistreptococcal interventions for guttate and chronic psoriasis. Br J Dermatol. 2001;145(6):886–90.
24. Fry L, Baker BS. Triggering psoriasis: the role of infections and medications. Clin Dermatol. 2007;25(6):606–15.
25. Tsankov N, Angelova I, Kazandjieva J. Drug-induced psoriasis. Recognition and management. Am J Clin Dermatol. 2000;1(3):159–65.
26. Piérard-Franchimont C, Piérard GE. Drug-related psoriasis. Rev Med Liege. 2012;67(3):139–42.
27. Balak DM, Hajdarbegovic E. Drug-induced psoriasis: clinical perspectives. Psoriasis (Auckl). 2017;7:87–94.
28. Kim GK, Del Rosso JQ. Drug-provoked psoriasis: is it drug induced or drug aggravated?: understanding pathophysiology and clinical relevance. J Clin Aesthet Dermatol. 2010;3(1):32–8.
29. Nestle FO, Conrad C, Tun-Kyi A, et al. Plasmacytoid predendritic cells initiate psoriasis through interferon-alpha production. J Exp Med. 2005;202(1):135–43.
30. Higgins E. Alcohol, smoking, and psoriasis. Clin Exp Dermatol. 2000;25(2):107–10.
31. Murzaku, EC, Bronsnick T, Rao BK. Diet in dermatology: part II. Melanoma, chronic urticaria, and psoriasis. J Am Acad Dermatol 2014, 71(6):1053.e1-1053.e16.
32. Poikolainen K, Karvonen J, Pukkala E. Excess mortality related to alcohol and smoking among hospital-treated patients with psoriasis. Arch Dermatol. 1999;135(12):1490–3.

33. Herron MD, Hinckley M, Hoffman MS, et al. Impact of obesity and smoking on psoriasis presentation and management. Arch Dermatol. 2005;141(12):1527–34.
34. Poikolainen K, Reunala T, Karvonen J. Smoking, alcohol and life events related to psoriasis among women. Br J Dermatol. 1994;130(4):473–7.
35. Naldi L, Chatenoud L, Linder D, et al. Cigarette smoking, body mass index, and stressful life events as risk factors for psoriasis: results from an Italian case-control study. J Invest Dermatol. 2005;125(1):61–7.
36. Tobin AM, Veale DJ, Fitzgerald O, et al. Cardiovascular disease and risk factors in patients with psoriasis and psoriatic arthritis. J Rheumatol. 2010;37(7):1386–94.
37. Fortes C, Mastroeni S, Leffondré K, et al. Relationship between smoking and the clinical severity of psoriasis. Arch Dermatol. 2005;141(12):1580–4.
38. Lee EJ, Han KD, Han JH, Lee JH. Smoking and risk of psoriasis: a nationwide cohort study. J Am Acad Dermatol. 2017;77(3):573–5.
39. Armstrong AW, Harskamp CT, Armstrong EJ. The association between psoriasis and obesity: a systematic review and meta-analysis of observational studies. Nutr Diabetes. 2012;2(12):e54.
40. Neimann AL, Shin DB, Wang X, Margolis DJ, Troxel AB, Gelfand JM. Prevalence of cardiovascular risk factors in patients with psoriasis. J Am Acad Dermatol. 2006;55(5):829–35.
41. Langan SM, Seminara NM, Shin DB, et al. Prevalence of metabolic syndrome in patients with psoriasis: a population-based study in the United Kingdom. J Invest Dermatol. 2012;132(3 Pt 1):556–62.
42. Cao H. Adipocytokines in obesity and metabolic disease. J Endocrinol. 2014;220(2):T47–59.
43. Versini M, Jeandel PY, Rosenthal E, Shoenfeld Y. Obesity in autoimmune diseases: not a passive bystander. Autoimmun Rev. 2014;13(9):981–1000.
44. Brembilla NC, Boehncke WH. Dermal adipocytes' claim for fame in psoriasis. Exp Dermatol. 2017;26(5):392–3.
45. Fortune DG, Richards HL, Griffiths CE. Psychologic factors in psoriasis: consequences, mechanisms, and interventions. Dermatol Clin. 2005;23(4):681–94.
46. Richards HL, Ray DW, Kirby B, et al. Response of the hypothalamic-pituitary-adrenal axis to psychological stress in patients with psoriasis. Br J Dermatol. 2005;153(6):1114–20.
47. Mowad CM, Margolis DJ, Halpern AC, Suri B, Synnestvedt M, Guzzo CA. Hormonal influences on women with psoriasis. Cutis. 1998;61(5):257–60.
48. Boehncke WH. Etiology and pathogenesis of psoriasis. Rheum Dis Clin N Am. 2015;41(4):665–75.
49. Di Meglio P, Villanova F, Nestle FO. Psoriasis. Cold Spring Harb Perspect Med. 2014;4(8):a015354.
50. Rendon A, Schäkel K. Psoriasis pathogenesis and treatment. Int J Mol Sci. 2019;20(6):1475.
51. Boehncke WH, Schön MP. Psoriasis. Lancet. 2015;386(9997):983–94.
52. Greb JE, Goldminz AM, Elder JT, Lebwohl MG, Gladman DD, Wu JJ, Mehta NN, Finlay AY, Gottlieb AB. Psoriasis. Nat Rev Dis Primers. 2016;24(2):16082.
53. Hugh JM, Weinberg JM. Update on the pathophysiology of psoriasis. Cutis. 2018;102(5S):6–12.
54. Benhadou F, Mintoff D, Del Marmol V. Psoriasis: keratinocytes or immune cells – which is the trigger? Dermatology. 2019;235(2):91–100.
55. Armstrong AW, Read C. Pathophysiology, clinical presentation, and treatment of psoriasis: a review. JAMA. 2020;323(19):1945–60.
56. Kirby B. Langerhans cells in psoriasis: getting to the core of the disease. Br J Dermatol. 2018;178(6):1240.
57. Gupta K, Harvima IT. Mast cell-neural interactions contribute to pain and itch. Immunol Rev. 2018;282(1):168–87.
58. Kim J, Krueger JG. The immunopathogenesis of psoriasis. Dermatol Clin. 2015;33(1):13–23.
59. Jariwala SP. The role of dendritic cells in the immunopathogenesis of psoriasis. Arch Dermatol Res. 2007;299(8):359–66.
60. Das RP, Jain AK, Ramesh V. Current concepts in the pathogenesis of psoriasis. Indian J Dermatol. 2009;54(1):7–12.

61. Ivanov II, Zhou L, Littman DR. Transcriptional regulation of Th17 cell differentiation. Semin Immunol. 2007;19(6):409–17.
62. Rose-John S. Interleukin-6 family cytokines. Cold Spring Harb Perspect Biol. 2018;10(2):a028415. Published 2018 Feb 1
63. Camporeale A, Poli V. IL-6, IL-17 and STAT3: a holy trinity in auto-immunity? Front Biosci (Landmark Ed). 2012;1(17):2306–26.
64. Mathur AN, Chang HC, Zisoulis DG, Stritesky GL, Yu Q, O'Malley JT, Kapur R, Levy DE, Kansas GS, Kaplan MH. Stat3 and Stat4 direct development of IL-17-secreting Th cells. J Immunol. 2007;178(8):4901–7.
65. Floss DM, Klöcker T, Schröder J, et al. Defining the functional binding sites of interleukin 12 receptor β1 and interleukin 23 receptor to Janus kinases. Mol Biol Cell. 2016;27(14):2301–16.
66. McGeachy MJ, Chen Y, Tato CM, et al. The interleukin 23 receptor is essential for the terminal differentiation of interleukin 17-producing effector T helper cells in vivo. Nat Immunol. 2009;10(3):314–24.
67. Dhar S, Banerjee R, Agrawal N, Chatterjee S, Malakar R. Psoriasis in children: an insight. Indian J Dermatol. 2011;56(3):262–5.

Clinical Features

Clinical manifestations of psoriasis in children include several and variable manifestations, related to the specific clinical type and to the severity of the disease.

Some clinical features of childhood psoriasis may sometimes make difficult the diagnosis of the disease in children, as clinical aspects could resemble other type of dermatitis as well as other skin diseases (such as atopic dermatitis, nummular eczema, seborrheic dermatitis, allergic and irritant contact dermatitis, skin infections) [1–3].

Most of patients (approximately 80% of children with psoriasis) have mild-to-moderate disease, although the commonly used severity scores evaluate only the clinical severity of psoriasis, often inducing to underestimate the percentage of patients with moderate-to-severe disease [1–4].

In fact, the most commonly parameters used in clinical studies to evaluate the severity of psoriasis include Body Surface Area (BSA), Psoriasis Area Severity Index (PASI), and Physicians Global Severity score; these parameters do not consider the different impact of the disease on the quality of life and on the general health of the patient related to the involvement of specific body areas.

The involvement of specific skin areas (such as face, genitals, hands) which are often exposed and visible may have a great impact on the quality of life of the patient, especially in children. In children and adolescents, the involvement of these areas is more common than in adults and could strongly influence family and social relationships with a great negative psychological impact on the child's quality of life.

Formal diagnostic criteria for psoriasis do not exist and diagnosis is based on the specific experience and clinical skills of the physician, also considering that in children the diagnosis of psoriasis is a clinical diagnosis as skin biopsy is not routinely performed on younger patients and should be reserved for the most difficult cases.

Laboratory investigations also have a limited role in the diagnosis of childhood psoriasis and should be considered only in particular forms (such as generalized

A. Belloni Fortina, F. Caroppo, *Pediatric Psoriasis*, https://doi.org/10.1007/978-3-030-90712-9_4

pustular psoriasis), in which a complete blood count, ionogram, and renal and hepatic function tests should be considered.

Therefore, it is important that dermatologists and pediatricians are able to recognize the principal clinical characteristics of psoriasis in children.

A clinical specific feature of psoriatic lesions, both in adults and children, is the "Auspitz sign" which consists in pinpoint bleeding after the removal of the scales by mechanical factors.

As in adults, also in children the most common clinical type of psoriasis overall is plaque psoriasis, which is characterized by sharply demarcated plaque with erythema and silvery scales [2–5].

However, psoriasis in children shows involvement of the face and anogenital regions more often than in adults, sometimes representing the unique manifestation of the disease.

In children there are some specific clinical features that delineate different clinical subtypes of childhood psoriasis (such as the frequent involvement of the face and flexural regions with thinner, smaller, less scaly lesions) (Table 4.1).

Furthermore, the typical thickened, scaly, erythematous, and well-demarcated plaques that are generally easy to recognize in adults are often absent and psoriatic plaques can resemble eczema in children [4–9] (Figs. 4.1, 4.2, 4.3, 4.4, and 4.5).

The clinical classification of childhood psoriasis is principally based on the shape, clinical aspect of the lesions, and on the involved body areas (Table 4.1).

In children some clinical subtypes of psoriasis, such as guttate and inverse psoriasis, are more common than in the adults.

Fig. 4.1 Plaque psoriasis in a child involving the lower limbs, with erythematous plaques covered by gray/silver lamellar scales and well-demarcated edges

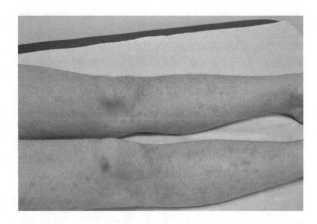

Fig. 4.2 Pediatric plaque psoriasis of the trunk

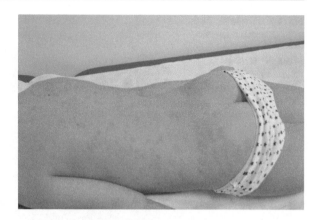

Fig. 4.3 Detail of a typical skin lesion of psoriasis in children: dry erythematous plaques covered by silver lamellar scales, with well-demarcated edges and a clear distinction between affected and non-affected skin areas

Fig. 4.4 Diffuse plaque psoriasis of the trunk in a 15-year-old boy

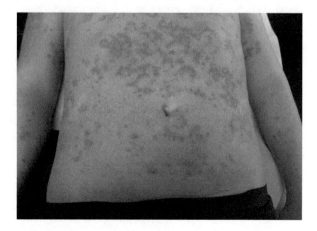

Fig. 4.5 Plaque psoriasis of the trunk in a 15-year-old boy. The typical lesions of plaque psoriasis in children are very thin plaques covered by gray-silver and fine scales, with well-demarcated edges

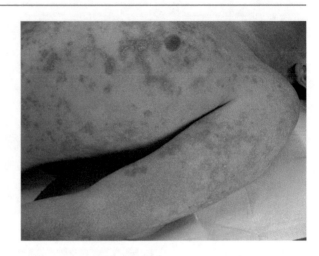

4.1 Clinical Types of Pediatric Psoriasis

4.1.1 Plaque Psoriasis

Plaque psoriasis is the most common form of the disease, not only in adults, but also in children. However, the prevalence of plaque psoriasis in children varies between 35 and 70%, while in adults the prevalence of plaque psoriasis is reported up to 90% [3, 5, 10–12].

Plaque-type psoriasis is clinically characterized by dry erythematous plaques covered by gray/silver lamellar scales. Plaques are typically monomorphic and show well-demarcated edges with a clear distinction between affected and non-affected skin areas.

Plaques of psoriasis can appear anywhere on the skin, but the most affected body areas in children are knees, elbows, scalp, face, post-auricular, umbilicus, and peri-umbilical region. Plaque psoriasis can also be itchy and generalized [2, 3, 5, 11–13] (Figs. 4.6, 4.7, 4.8, 4.9, 4.10, 4.11, 4.12, 4.13, 4.14, 4.15, 4.16, 4.17, 4.18, 4.19, 4.20, 4.21, and 4.22).

Skin lesions of plaque-type psoriasis in children usually are smaller, thinner and with less flaking compared with psoriatic lesions in adults.

Table 4.1 Clinical subtypes of psoriasis

Clinical subtype of psoriasis	Main characteristics	Localization of skin lesions
Plaque psoriasis	• The most common type in children (prevalence in children: 35–70%) • Clinically characterized by dry erythematous plaques covered by gray/silver lamellar scales, with well-demarcated edges and a clear distinction between affected and non-affected skin areas	• Knees, elbows, scalp, face, limbs, post-auricular regions, umbilicus, periumbilical region
Scalp psoriasis	• Common clinical subtype of psoriasis in children and adolescents, affecting up to 79% of the patients • Scalp psoriasis tends to be more common in girls than in boys. Often represents the first location at the onset of the disease • Clinically characterized by thick, adherent silver/white scales, sometimes appearing as "pityriasis amiantacea" with encasing of the hair shaft and a possible temporary hair loss	• Scalp, extending to the forehead, over the ears and on the nape of the neck
Guttate psoriasis	• More common in children than in adults (30% of the total cases of childhood psoriasis) • Clinically characterized by a widespread acute eruption with small (<1 cm), drop-like erythematous or red-to-salmon scaly dot-shaped papules or plaques with fine desquamation • Guttate psoriasis is the clinical subtype most commonly related to a previous infection as trigger factor (often preceded by a group A beta hemolytic streptococcus infection of the upper respiratory tract in the most of cases and, less frequently, of other body areas) • In children seems more common in subjects with a positive familial history of psoriasis and in patients with moderate-to-severe than mild disease	• Trunk, extremities, face, scalp
Inverse psoriasis	• More common in children than in adults • Clinically characterized by erythematous, bright-red plaques with well-defined edges. The plaques appear usually dry, glazed and without or few scales • The typical absence or reduced desquamation of the inverse psoriasis' lesions is usually related to the most common moisture and maceration of these areas, where lesions may be associated with secondary infections by Candida or streptococcus • The frequency of involvement of anogenital regions generally decreases with increasing age of the child and inverse psoriasis later tends to present in other body areas or with more typical lesions of the classic plaque-type psoriasis	• The most affected areas are the flexural and intertriginous regions, including axillae, retro-auricular regions, inguinal folds, and genital or perianal areas • In infants the most frequent clinical type of psoriasis is a particular form of inverse psoriasis related to the involvement of diaper area ("napkin psoriasis")

(continued)

Table 4.1 (continued)

Clinical subtype of psoriasis	Main characteristics	Localization of skin lesions
Palmoplantar psoriasis	• Prevalence in children ranges from 10% to 20%, with a higher frequency in children under 12 years of age • The clinical characteristics of the lesions of palmoplantar psoriasis are usually related to the classic plaque-type psoriasis, with well-demarcated edges between affected and non-affected areas	• Palmoplantar regions
Nail psoriasis	• Children with psoriasis show nail involvement in 30–40% of cases, with a higher prevalence in male children • Nail involvement could be the first and unique sign of psoriasis in children • Clinically usually characterized by pitting, onycholysis, and pachyonychia, with a major prevalence of onycholysis and pachyonychia in toenails. Beau lines, discoloration with yellow and brownish patches, leukonychia, paronychia, and splinter hemorrhages are other possible clinical characteristics of nail psoriasis • As in adults, also in children, nail psoriasis is more frequently associated with psoriasis arthritis compared to the other clinical subtypes of psoriasis	• Fingernails and/or toenails
Pustular psoriasis	• A less common variant of childhood psoriasis • Clinically characterized by sterile superficial and coalescing pustules • Annular configuration of pustules is most common in children than in adults • Disseminated pustular psoriasis may be associated with systemic involvement, with fever and malaise, and could be life threatening	• Disseminated or localized (trunk, limbs, palmoplantar regions)
Follicular psoriasis	• A rare variant of childhood psoriasis although probably under-diagnosed • Clinically characterized by discrete hyperkeratotic papules and follicular lesions with a grouped and asymmetrical distribution	• Localized in grouped and asymmetrical distribution, involving the trunk, thighs, axillae, and bony prominences
Erythrodermic psoriasis	• A rare clinical subtype of psoriasis in children and in adults • Clinically characterized by a generalized involvement of the skin (more than 90% of the body surface area) with a generalized erythema and scarce scaling • Possible presence of pustules or blisters • Frequent itch and/or pain • Possible increase of body temperature • Represents a life-threatening variant with systemic symptoms, such as fever and general malaise	• Generalized

Fig. 4.6 Severe plaque
psoriasis of the trunk in a
14-year-old boy

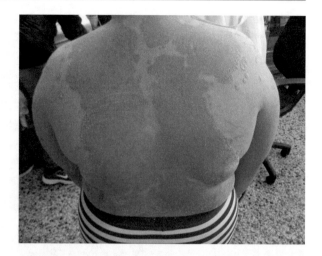

Fig. 4.7 Severe plaque
psoriasis of the trunk in a
14-year-old boy

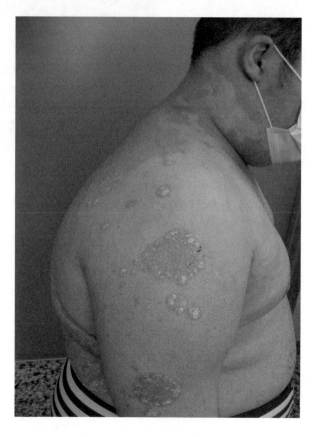

Fig. 4.8 Plaque psoriasis
of the elbows in a
14-year-old boy

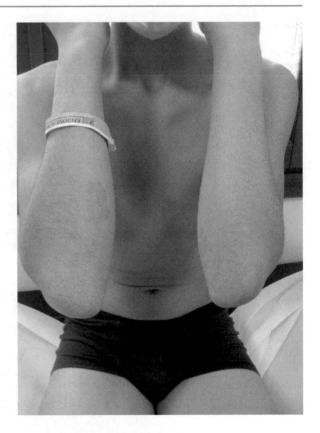

Fig. 4.9 Plaque psoriasis
of the elbows in a
13-year-old girl

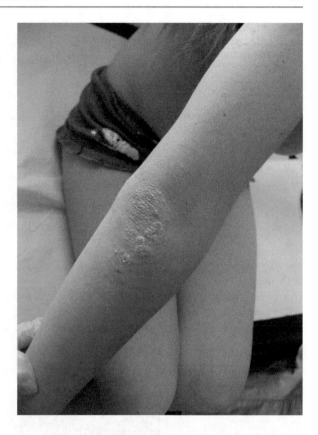

Fig. 4.10 Plaque psoriasis
of the trunk

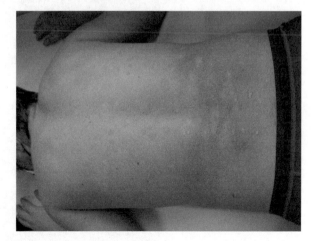

Fig. 4.11 Plaque psoriasis
involving the neck, scalp,
and face in a young girl

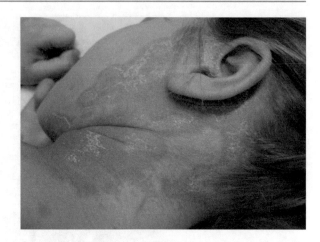

Fig. 4.12 Plaque psoriasis
of the trunk

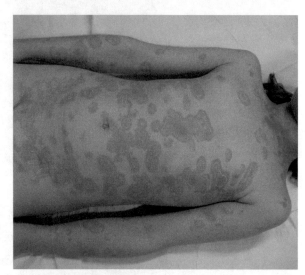

Fig 4.13 Plaque psoriasis
of the trunk in a young
female child with
erythematous figurate
lesions

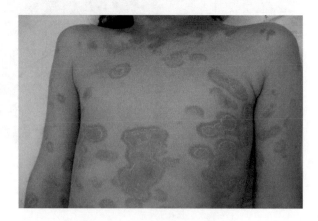

Fig. 4.14 Plaque psoriasis extending on the neck and face

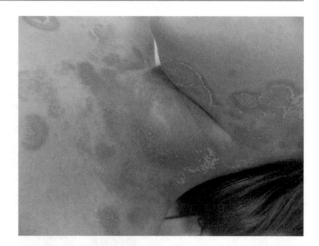

Fig. 4.15 Severe plaque psoriasis in a girl involving all the body area

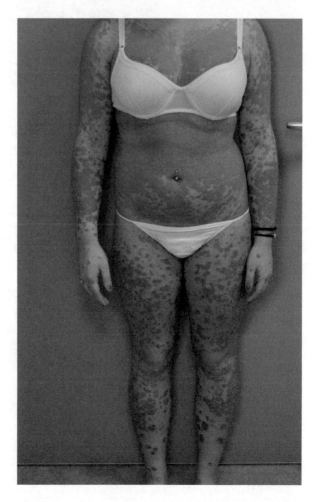

Fig. 4.16 Severe plaque
psoriasis in a girl involving
all the body area

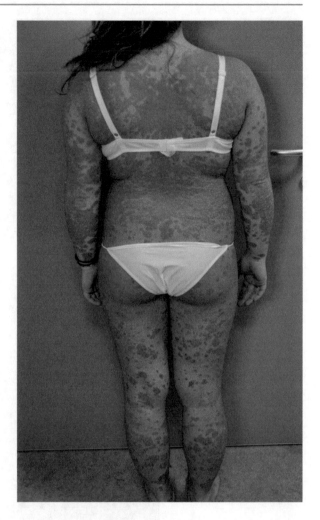

Fig. 4.17 Psoriatic skin
lesions of the elbows in
a girl

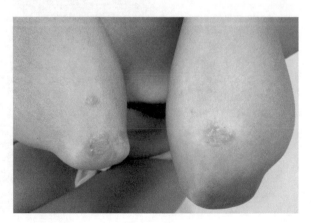

Fig. 4.18 Plaque psoriasis of the trunk in a child

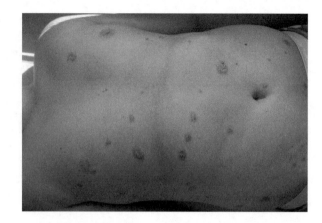

Fig. 4.19 Psoriatic skin lesions of the knees in a child

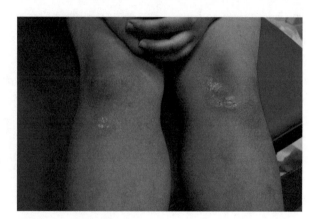

Fig. 4.20 Psoriatic skin lesions of the knees in a child

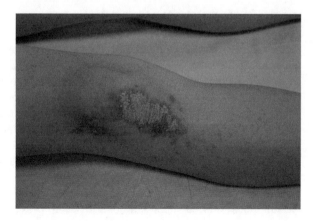

Fig. 4.21 Plaque psoriasis of the trunk in a young male child

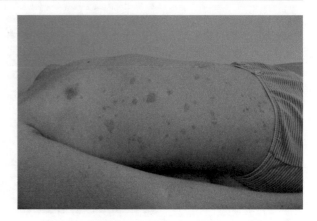

Fig. 4.22 Plaque psoriasis of the trunk in a young male child

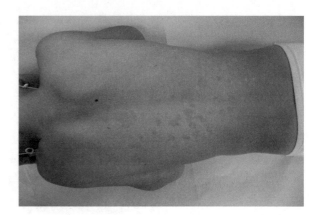

4.1.2   Scalp Psoriasis

Scalp psoriasis is a common clinical subtype of psoriasis in children and adolescents, affecting up to 79% of the patients [2, 3, 5, 10, 12].

In girls scalp psoriasis tends to be more common than in boys and in many children, scalp psoriasis represents the first location at the onset of the disease.

Scalp psoriasis is clinically characterized by erythematous patches and plaques of skin covered by thick, adherent silver/white scales, sometimes appearing as "pityriasis amiantacea" with encasing of the hair shaft and with a possible temporary hair loss in the affected areas (Figs. 4.23, 4.24, 4.25, 4.26, 4.27, 4.28, 4.29, 4.30, 4.31, 4.32, 4.33, 4.34, 4.35, and 4.36).

Scalp psoriasis can be mild and sometimes unnoticeable, but it can also be severe, causing thick, crusted sores. Furthermore, scalp psoriasis may be intensely itchy,

Fig. 4.23 Mild scalp psoriasis in a child with thin erythematous patches covered by adherent silver/white scales

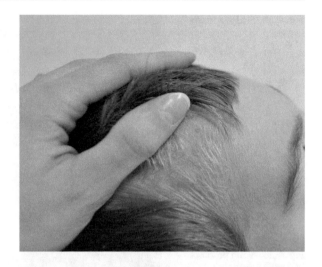

Fig. 4.24 Mild scalp psoriasis in a child with thin erythematous patches covered by adherent silver/white scales

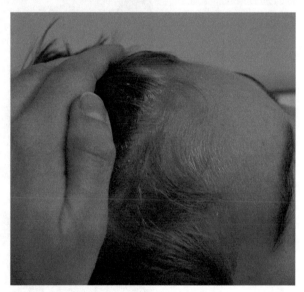

with a consequent possible negative impact on quality of life of the patient and the risk of skin infections due to scratching [2, 3, 5, 10, 12].

4.1.3   Guttate Psoriasis

Guttate psoriasis (or "drop-like" psoriasis) is more common in children and adolescents than in adults, affecting up to 30% of cases of childhood psoriasis, still remaining the second most common clinical type of psoriasis overall [14, 15].

Fig. 4.25 Scalp psoriasis
in a child

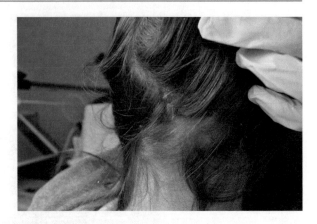

Fig. 4.26 Scalp psoriasis
in a child involving neck
and retroauricular regions

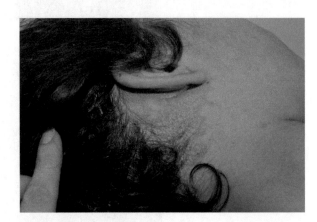

Fig. 4.27 Detail of a
typical skin lesion of scalp
psoriasis of a child

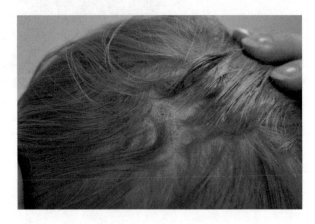

Fig. 4.28 Detail of the typical skin lesion of scalp psoriasis in a child

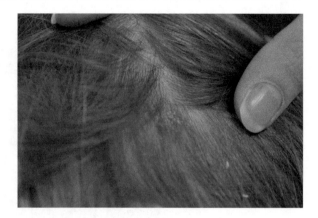

Fig. 4.29 Psoriasis in a female child involving scalp and retroauricular regions

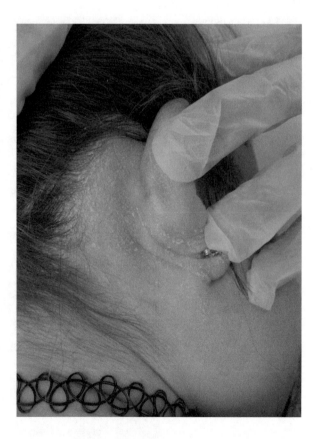

Fig. 4.30 Scalp psoriasis in a female child

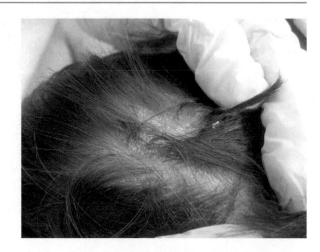

Fig. 4.31 Scalp psoriasis in a female child

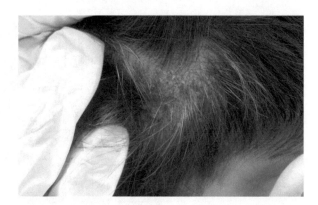

Fig. 4.32 Scalp psoriasis in a young female child

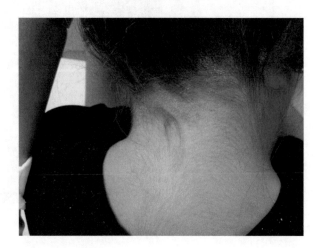

Fig. 4.33 Detail of a typical skin lesion of scalp psoriasis in a child

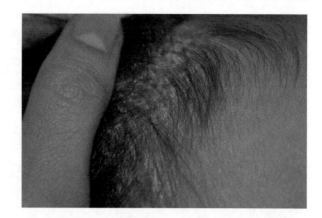

Fig. 4.34 Detail of a typical skin lesion of scalp psoriasis in a child

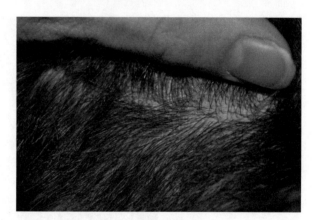

Fig. 4.35 Detail of a typical skin lesion of scalp psoriasis in a child

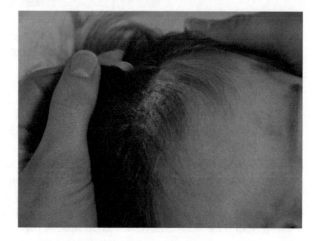

Fig. 4.36 Detail of a typical skin lesion of scalp psoriasis in a child

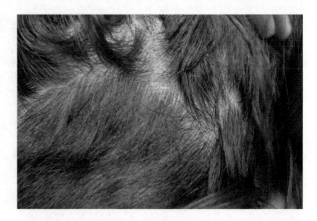

Fig. 4.37 Guttate psoriasis in a young child with widespread acute eruption with small, drop-like erythematous/red-to-salmon scaly dot-shaped papules and plaques with fine desquamation

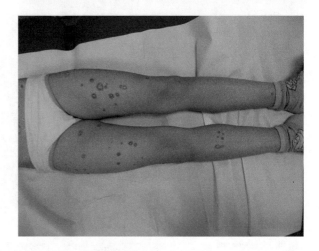

Guttate psoriasis is clinically characterized by a widespread acute eruption with small (usually less than 1 cm), dot-shaped, red-to-salmon colored plaques with fine desquamation.

The lesions of guttate psoriasis are usually diffuse, with a most common involvement of the trunk, abdomen, and back (Figs. 4.37, 4.38, 4.39, 4.40, 4.41, and 4.42).

Although guttate psoriasis usually resolves within 4–5 months, in one-third of children guttate psoriasis persists evolving into a classic plaque-type form in later life [14–16].

Among the different clinical subtypes of psoriasis, guttate psoriasis is the most commonly form related to a previous infection as principal recognized trigger factor. In particular, guttate psoriasis is often preceded by a group A beta hemolytic streptococcus infection of the upper respiratory tract in the most of cases and, less frequently, of other body areas (such as perianal or vulvar regions) [3, 5, 10, 15, 16].

Fig. 4.38 Guttate
psoriasis in a young child

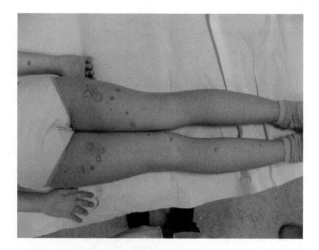

Fig. 4.39 Guttate
psoriasis in a young child
involving the trunk

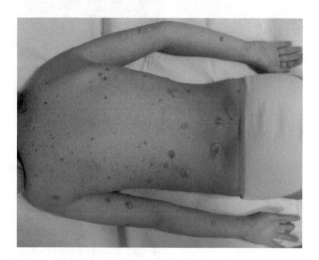

Several data suggest that in children with guttate psoriasis related to a streptococcus infection, the disease can spontaneously resolve, while in patients without
streptococcus infection as trigger factor, the disease can persist, evolving to a
chronic plaque-type psoriasis.

Guttate psoriasis in children seems more common in subjects with a positive
familial history of psoriasis and in patients with moderate-to-severe than mild disease [10, 15, 16].

Fig. 4.40 Guttate
psoriasis in a male child

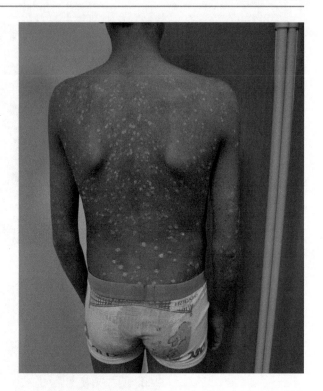

Fig. 4.41 Guttate
psoriasis in a male child

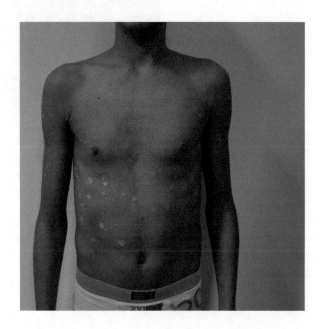

Fig. 4.42 Guttate psoriasis of the trunk in a young child

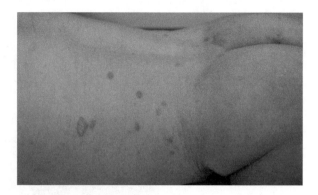

Fig. 4.43 Inverse psoriasis of the axillae in a young female child with the typical skin lesions: erythematous, bright-red plaques with well-defined edges, usually dry, glazed and without or few scales

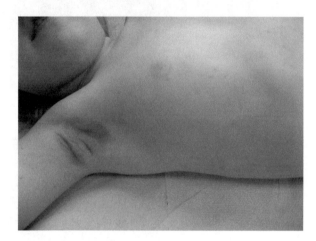

4.1.4   Inverse Psoriasis

Inverse psoriasis is more common in children than in adults, affecting most frequently infants and young children.

The most affected areas are the flexural and intertriginous regions, including axillae, retro-auricular regions, inguinal folds, and genital or perianal areas; in infants the most frequent clinical type of psoriasis is a specific form of inverse psoriasis related to the involvement of diaper area, delineating the specific clinical subtype of "napkin psoriasis." [3, 5, 10, 15, 17] (Figs. 4.43, 4.44, 4.45, 4.46, 4.47, 4.48, 4.49, 4.50, 4.51, 4.52, 4.53, 4.54, 4.55, 4.56, 4.57, and 4.58).

Inverse psoriasis is clinically characterized by erythematous, bright-red plaques with well-defined edges. The plaques appear usually dry, glazed and without or few scales (Figs. 4.43, 4.44, 4.45, 4.46, 4.47, 4.48, 4.49, 4.50, 4.51, 4.52, 4.53, 4.54, 4.55, 4.56, 4.57, and 4.58).

Therefore, sometimes it can be difficult to distinguish napkin psoriasis from other common napkin rashes; so in these cases it would be helpful to investigate

Fig. 4.44 Inverse psoriasis involving the inguinal folds in a child

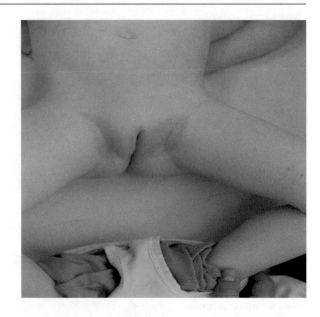

Fig. 4.45 Inverse psoriasis involving axillae in a male infant

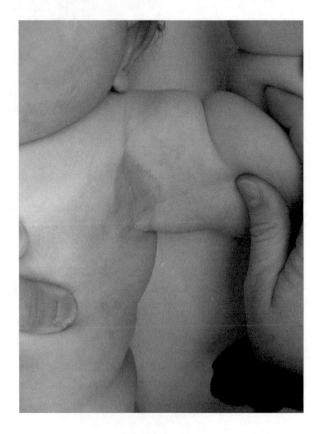

Fig. 4.46 Inverse psoriasis involving the neck in a male infant

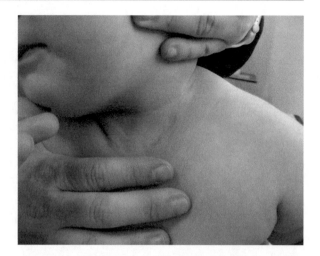

Fig. 4.47 Inverse psoriasis involving genital region in a male adolescent

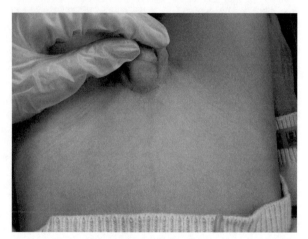

Fig. 4.48 Inverse psoriasis involving axillae and antecubital folds in an infant

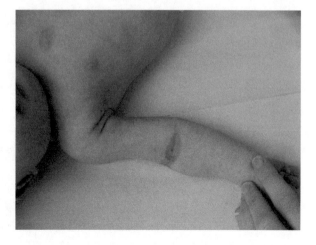

Fig. 4.49 Detail of the
typical skin lesions of
inverse psoriasis:
erythematous, bright-red
plaques with well-defined
edges, usually dry, glazed
and without or few scales

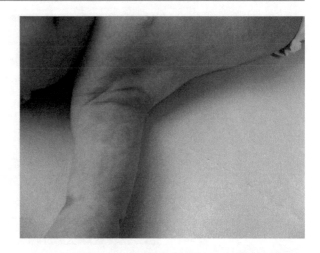

Fig. 4.50 Typical inverse
psoriasis of the infant
involving inguinal folds
("napkin psoriasis").
Napkin psoriasis in infants
should be differentiated
from irritant napkin
dermatitis investigating the
involvement of the entire
fold areas, which is typical
of napkin psoriasis and is
usually absent in irritant
napkin dermatitis

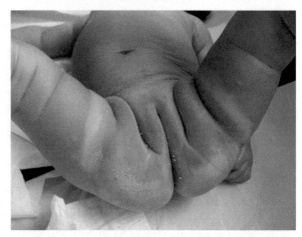

Fig. 4.51 Inverse
psoriasis of the infant
involving inguinal folds
("napkin psoriasis")

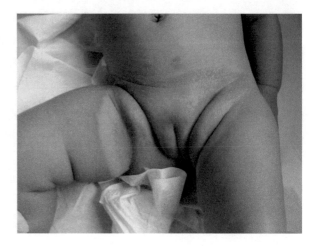

Fig. 4.52 Inverse
psoriasis of the infant
("napkin psoriasis")

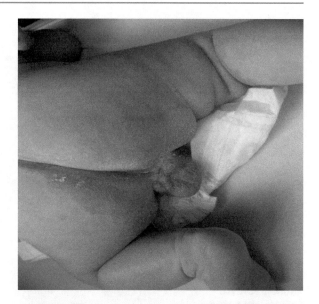

Fig. 4.53 Inverse
psoriasis of the infant
("napkin psoriasis")

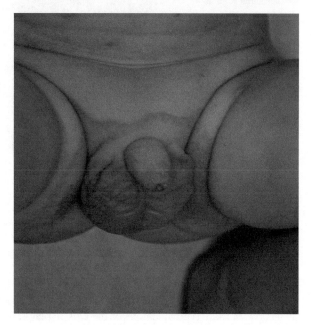

lesions of inverse psoriasis in other body regions (such as other flexural areas, axillae, umbilical region) or lesions related to plaque-type psoriasis [10, 15, 17].

Furthermore, diaper psoriasis in infants should be differentiated from irritant napkin dermatitis investigating the involvement of the entire fold areas, which is typical of napkin psoriasis and is usually absent in irritant napkin dermatitis.

Fig. 4.54 Inverse
psoriasis of the infant
involving neck

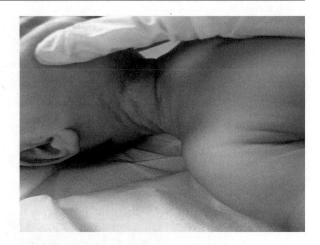

Fig. 4.55 Inverse
psoriasis of the infant
involving neck and
retroauricular regions

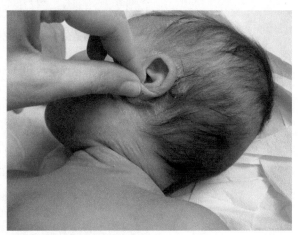

The typical absence or reduced desquamation of the inverse psoriasis' lesions is usually related to the most common moisture and maceration of these areas, where lesions may be associated with secondary infections by Candida or Streptococcus, especially in infants with napkin psoriasis, requiring topical anti-infective drugs or specific skin cultures [10, 15, 16].

The frequency of involvement of anogenital regions generally decreases with increasing age of the child and inverse psoriasis later tends to present in other body areas or with more typical lesions of the classic plaque-type psoriasis.

4.1.5   Palmoplantar Psoriasis

Palmoplantar psoriasis defines a specific subtype of psoriasis characterized by the involvement of palmoplantar regions [2, 3, 5, 15].

Fig. 4.56 Inverse psoriasis of the infant

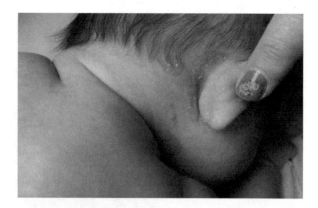

Fig. 4.57 Inverse psoriasis in a child

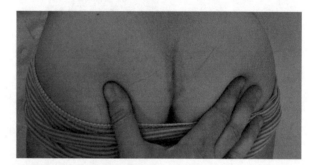

Fig. 4.58 Inverse psoriasis of the infant involving axillae

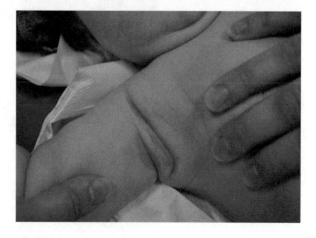

Prevalence of palmoplantar involvement in children with psoriasis ranges from 10 to 20%, with a higher frequency in children under 12 years of age [15–18].

The clinical characteristics of the lesions of palmoplantar psoriasis are usually related to the classic plaque-type psoriasis, with well-demarcated edges between affected and non-affected areas. In a minority of cases, the lesions are related to the pustular type psoriasis (Figs. 4.59, 4.60, 4.61, 4.62, 4.63, 4.64, 4.65, and 4.66).

Fig. 4.59 Palmoplantar
psoriasis in a child with
typical skin lesions: classic
plaque-type psoriasis, with
well-demarcated edges
between affected and
non-affected areas

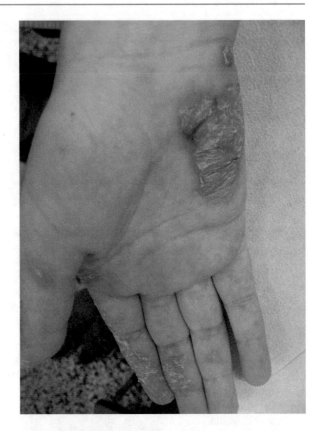

Fig. 4.60 Palmoplantar
psoriasis in a child with
typical skin lesions
involving palms

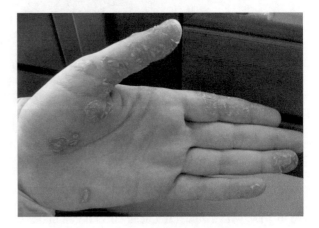

Fig. 4.61 Palmoplantar
psoriasis in a child

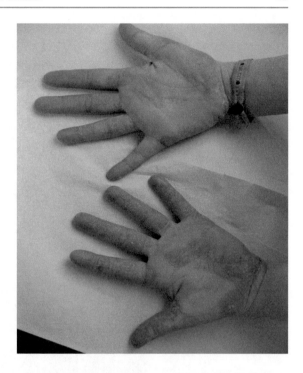

Fig. 4.62 Palmoplantar
psoriasis in a child

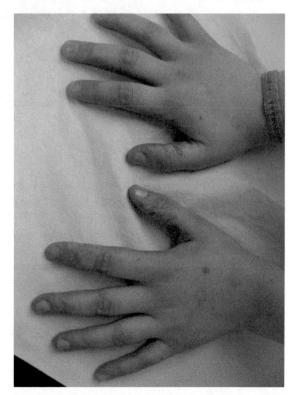

Fig. 4.63 Palmoplantar
psoriasis in a child

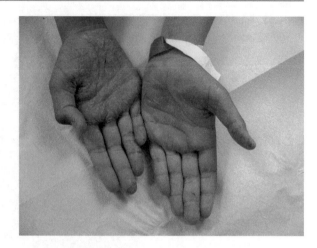

Fig. 4.64 Palmoplantar
psoriasis involving plantar
regions in a child

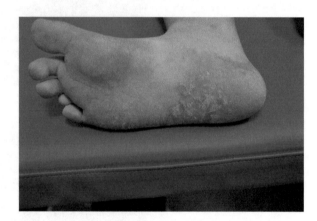

4.1.6   Nail Psoriasis

Children with psoriasis show nail involvement in 30-40% of cases, with a higher
prevalence in male children. Sometimes nail involvement could be the first and
unique sign of psoriasis in children.

Nail psoriasis is clinically usually characterized by pitting, onycholysis, and
pachyonychia, with a major prevalence of onycholysis and pachyonychia in toe-
nails. Beau lines, discoloration with yellow and brownish patches, leukonychia,
paronychia, and splinter hemorrhages are other possible clinical characteristics of
nail psoriasis [2, 3, 5, 10, 13, 19] (Figs. 4.65, 4.66, 4.67, 4.68, 4.69, 4.70, 4.71, 4.72,
4.73, and 4.74).

As in adults, nail pediatric psoriasis is more frequently associated with psoriasis
arthritis compared to the other clinical subtypes of psoriasis, as a result of the

Fig. 4.65 Palmoplantar psoriasis in a child involving hands and finger nails

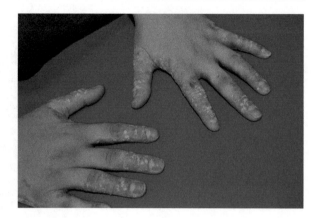

Fig. 4.66 Detail of the psoriatic skin lesions in a palmoplantar psoriasis involving fingers and nails

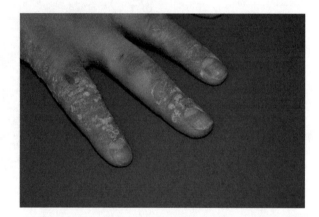

Fig. 4.67 Nail psoriasis in a young male child with typical clinical characteristics (pitting, discoloration with yellow and brownish patches, leukonychia, paronychia)

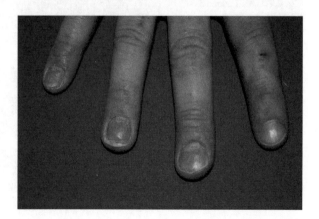

Fig. 4.68 Nail psoriasis in a child with typical clinical findings (pitting, trachyonichia, onycholysis, pachyonychia, discoloration with yellow and brownish patches, leukonychia)

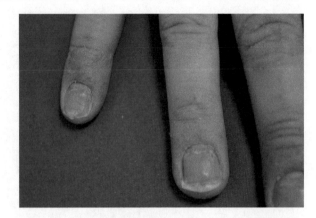

Fig. 4.69 Psoriasis of the nail showing with pitting, onycholysis, and pachyonychia

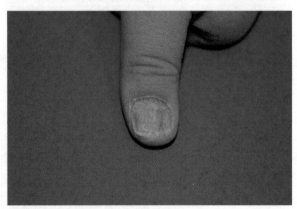

Fig. 4.70 Nail psoriasis of toe nails in a child

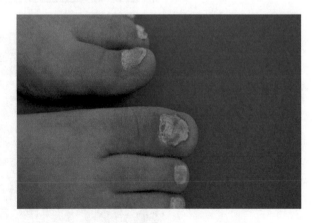

Fig. 4.71   Nail psoriasis of
toe nails in a child

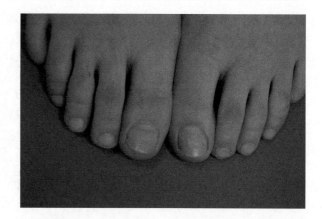

Fig. 4.72   Nail psoriasis in
a female child

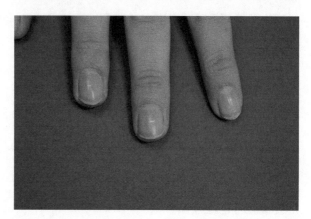

Fig. 4.73   Detail of
involvement of finger nails
in nail psoriasis

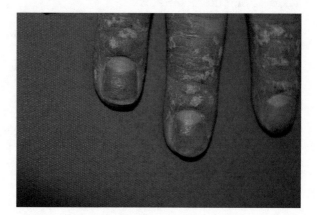

Fig. 4.74 Nail psoriasis

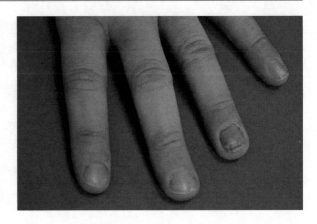

involvement of distal interphalangeal joints and nail matrix with the probable consequent enthesopathy.

4.1.7   Pustular Psoriasis

Pustular psoriasis is a less common variant of childhood psoriasis, clinically characterized by sterile superficial and coalescing pustules.

An annular configuration of pustules is most common in children than in adults (Figs. 4.75, 4.76, 4.77, 4.78, and 4.79).

The lesions could be localized or generalized. Disseminated pustular psoriasis may be associated with systemic involvement, with fever and malaise, and could be life threatening [2, 3, 5].

4.1.8   Follicular Psoriasis

Although in literature few data are reported about the clinical type of follicular psoriasis, this is a not uncommon variant.

The diagnosis of follicular psoriasis is probably underestimated due to a lack of awareness by dermatologists, both in adults and in children. However, follicular psoriasis is commonly reported in pediatric age [20–24].

Follicular psoriasis is clinically characterized by discrete hyperkeratotic papules and follicular lesions commonly affecting the trunk, thighs, axillae, and bony prominences with a grouped and asymmetrical distribution [23, 24] (Figs. 4.80, 4.81, and 4.82).

Fig. 4.75 Disseminated pustular psoriasis in a male child with typical skin lesions (sterile superficial and coalescing pustules)

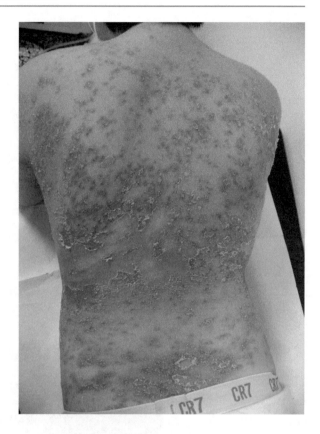

Fig. 4.76 Disseminated pustular psoriasis in a male child with typical skin lesions (sterile superficial and coalescing pustules)

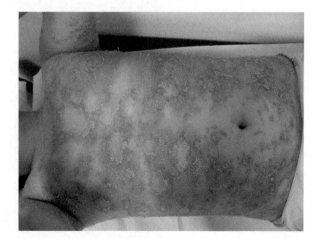

Fig. 4.77 Disseminated pustular psoriasis in a male child

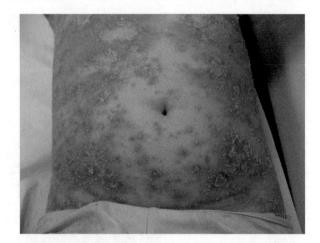

Fig. 4.78 Pustular psoriasis in a male child

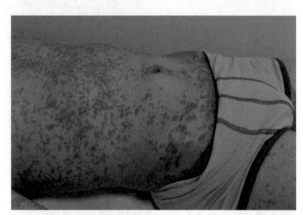

Fig. 4.79 Pustular psoriasis in a male child

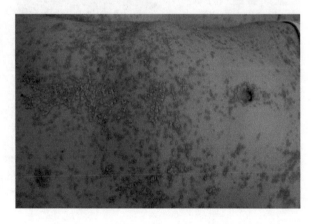

Fig. 4.80 Follicular psoriasis in a young male child with typical discrete hyperkeratotic papules and follicular lesions involving knees and lower limbs

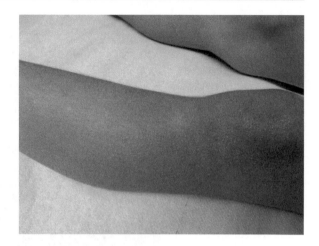

Fig. 4.81 Follicular psoriasis in a young male child with typical discrete hyperkeratotic papules and follicular lesions involving back of hands

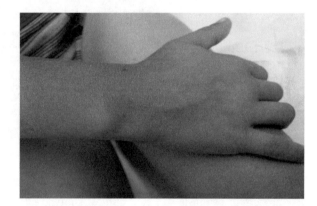

Fig. 4.82 Follicular psoriasis in a young male child with typical discrete hyperkeratotic papules and follicular lesions involving knees and lower limbs

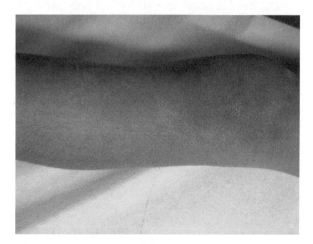

Fig. 4.83 Erythrodermic psoriasis in a male adolescent with a generalized involvement of the skin (more than 90% of the body surface area) and a generalized erythema and scarce scaling

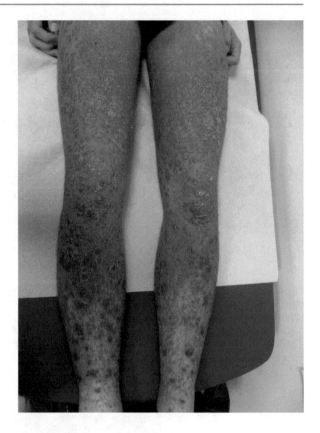

4.1.9   Erythrodermic Psoriasis

Erythrodermic psoriasis is a rare clinical subtype of psoriasis in children and in adults. Erythrodermic psoriasis is clinically characterized by a generalized involvement of the skin (more than 90% of the body surface area) with a generalized erythema and scarce scaling. Pustules or blisters may also be present, and itch or pain are symptoms commonly associated (Figs. 4.83, 4.84, 4.85, 4.86, 4.87, and 4.88).

Erythrodermic psoriasis is a rare, but serious condition and represents a life-threatening variant with systemic symptoms, such as fever and general malaise [2, 3, 5, 10].

In doubtful cases, a skin biopsy should be done in order to rule out cutaneous T-cell lymphomas.

Fig. 4.84 Erythrodermic
psoriasis in a male
adolescent

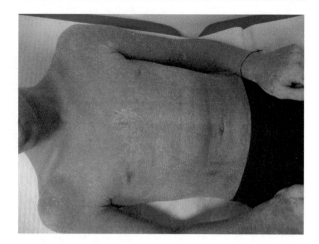

Fig. 4.85 Erythrodermic
psoriasis in a male
adolescent

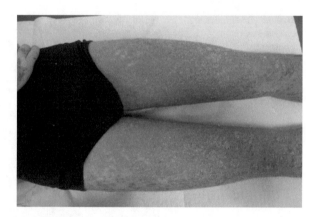

Fig. 4.86 Erythrodermic
psoriasis in a male
adolescent

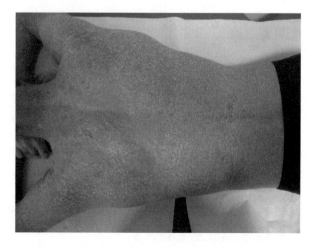

Fig. 4.87 Erythrodermic psoriasis in a male adolescent

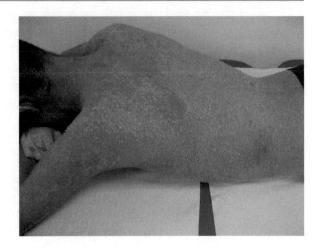

Fig. 4.88 Erythrodermic psoriasis in a male adolescent

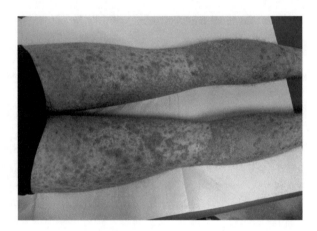

References

1. Megna M, Napolitano M, Balato A, et al. Psoriasis in children: a review. Curr Pediatr Rev. 2015;11(1):10–26.
2. Relvas M, Torres T. Pediatric psoriasis. Am J Clin Dermatol. 2017;18(6):797–811.
3. Mahé E. Childhood psoriasis. Eur J Dermatol. 2016;26(6):537–48.
4. Forward E, Lee G, Fischer G. Shades of grey: what is paediatric psoriasiform dermatitis and what does it have in common with childhood psoriasis? Clin Exp Dermatol. 2021;46(1):65–73.
5. Eichenfield LF, Paller AS, Tom WL, et al. Pediatric psoriasis: evolving perspectives. Pediatr Dermatol. 2018;35(2):170–81.
6. Seyhan M, Coskun BK, Saglam H, et al. Psoriasis in childhood and adolescence: evaluation of demographic and clinical features. Pediatr Int. 2006;48:525–30.
7. Barisic-Drusko V, Rucevic I. Psoriasis in childhood. Coll Anthropol. 2004;1:211–85.
8. Eickstaedt JB, Killpack L, Tung J, et al. Psoriasis and psoriasiform eruptions in pediatric patients with inflammatory bowel disease treated with anti–tumor necrosis factor alpha agents. Pediatr Dermatol. 2017;34:253–60.

9. Boehncke WH, Schon MP. Psoriasis. Lancet. 2015;386(9997):983–94.
10. Silverberg NB. Update on pediatric psoriasis, part 1: clinical features and demographics. Cutis. 2010;86(3):118–24.
11. Howard R, Tsuchiya A. Adult skin disease in the pediatric patient. Dermatol Clin. 1998;16(3):593–608.
12. Mercy K, Kwasny M, Cordoro KM, et al. Clinical manifestations of pediatric psoriasis: results of a multicenter study in the United States. Pediatr Dermatol. 2013;30(4):424–8.
13. Reich K. Approach to managing patients with nail psoriasis. J Eur Acad Dermatol Venereol. 2009;23(Suppl. 1):15–21.
14. Honig PJ. Guttate psoriasis associated with perianal streptococcal disease. J Pediatr. 1988;113(6):1037–9.
15. Tollefson MM. Diagnosis and management of psoriasis in children. Pediatr Clin N Am. 2014;61(2):261–77.
16. Bronckers IM, Paller AS, van Geel MJ, van de Kerkhof PC, Seyger MM. Psoriasis in children and adolescents: diagnosis. Management and comorbidities. Paediatr Drugs. 2015;17(5):373–84.
17. Mortz CG, Brockow K, Bindslev-Jensen C, Broesby-Olsen S. It looks like childhood eczema but is it? Clin Exp Allergy. 2019;49(6):744–53.
18. Morris A, Rogers M, Fischer G, Williams K. Childhood psoriasis: a clinical review of 1262 cases. Pediatr Dermatol. 2001;18:188–98.
19. Pinson R, Sotoodian B, Fiorillo L. Psoriasis in children. Psoriasis (Auckl). 2016;6:121–9.
20. Cordoro KM. Management of childhood psoriasis. Adv Dermatol. 2008;28:125–69.
21. Benoit S, Hamm H. Childhood psoriasis. Clin Dermatol. 2007;25(6):555–62.
22. Griffiths CE, Barker JN. Pathogenesis and clinical features of psoriasis. Lancet. 2007;370(9583):263–71.
23. Souza BCE, Bandeira LG, Cunha TDAC, Valente NYS. Follicular psoriasis: an underdiagnosed entity? An Bras Dermatol. 2019;94(1):116–8.
24. Shah KN. Diagnosis and treatment of pediatric psoriasis: current and future. Am J Clin Dermatol. 2013;14(3):195–213.

Diagnosis

5

In almost one-third of cases, psoriasis begins during childhood and adolescence and its appearance in pediatric age has several and variable manifestations, related to the specific clinical types and to the severity of the disease.

Most of children with psoriasis (approximately 80%) have mild to moderate disease and the lesions of psoriasis in children are generally thinner, smaller, less scaly compared to adults [1–5].

Therefore, the diagnosis of childhood psoriasis could be more challenging when compared to the well-delineated psoriasis in adults, also considering that formal diagnostic criteria for psoriasis do not exist and that diagnosis is primarily based on the clinical features of skin lesions (Fig. 5.1).

Skin biopsy is rarely performed on younger patients and should be reserved for the most difficult or doubtful cases, so a correct diagnosis of psoriasis often depends on the specific experience and clinical skills of the dermatologist or pediatrician [6–12].

Histological findings of the skin affected by psoriasis commonly include hyperkeratosis, parakeratosis (persistence of nucleated keratinocytes in the stratum corneum), epidermal acanthosis, absence or reduction of the granular cell layer, presence of a mixed perivascular inflammatory infiltrates, and edema of the papillary dermis with dilated blood vessels [7–16].

Two possible pathognomonic findings in psoriasis histology are the spongiform pustule of Kogoj and the microabscess of Munro: pustules of Kogoj are neutrophilic spongiotic aggregates in the stratum spinosum, while microabscess of Munro is characterized by the presence of neutrophils in the stratum corneum. On dermoscopy, dotted vessels can be seen in psoriatic plaques [8–16].

About clinical manifestations of psoriasis, although there are several sub-clinical types of disease in pediatric age, some clinical findings are characteristic of psoriasis both in adults and in children, such as the "Koebner phenomenon" (the appearance of new skin lesions after mechanical trauma on previously unaffected skin areas), the "Auspitz sign" (spots pinpoint bleeding after the removal of the scales by

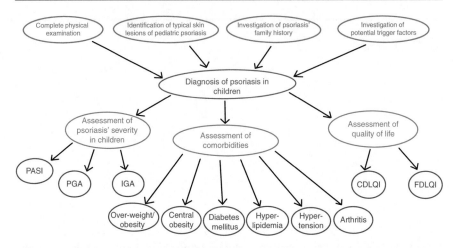

Fig. 5.1 Diagram about diagnostic process of childhood psoriasis and the assessment of disease's severity, comorbidities, and quality of life in children. *PASI* Psoriasis Area Severity Index, *PGA* Physician Global Assessment, *IGA* Investigator Global Assessment, *CDLQI* Children's Dermatology Life Quality Index, *FDLQI* Family Dermatology Life Quality Index

Fig. 5.2 Appearance of psoriatic skin lesions on previously unaffected skin areas in a child in the contact area with glasses ("Koebner phenomenon")

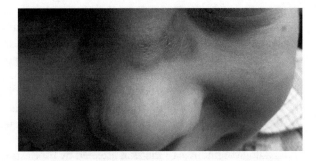

mechanical factors) and the presence of post-inflammatory pigmentary skin alterations (Figs. 5.2 and 5.3) [7–16].

Plaque psoriasis is the most common clinical subtype of psoriasis both in adults and in children and in this clinical subtype, the typical well-defined psoriatic lesions are generally found on the extensor surfaces of the limbs, but also on the scalp, face, and trunk.

However, some clinical subtypes (such as scalp, guttate, and inverse psoriasis) and the involvement of the scalp, face, and anogenital regions are more common in children.

In children, scalp psoriasis is clinically characterized by erythematous and hyperkeratotic patches and plaques of skin covered by thick, adherent silver/white scales, sometimes appearing as "pityriasis amiantacea" with encasing of the hair shaft and with a possible temporary hair loss in the affected areas. Pityriasis ami-antacea is typical of childhood and is considered by some authors a form of *"de*

Fig. 5.3 Onset of a psoriatic lesion in the contact area of the bra hook in a young girl ("Koebner phenomenon")

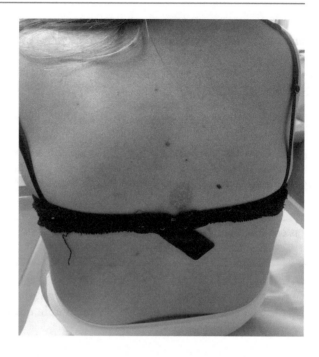

facto psoriasis," often representing the unique localization of the disease without any other specific clinical signs [1–9].

The history and clinical features of childhood psoriasis could also differ depending on the age of the child and on the clinical subtype of disease; for example, infants with psoriasis often show a persistent diaper rash that has been refractory to several topical therapies.

Besides the specific several clinical features of psoriasis in children, in the diagnostic process a special attention should be given to the familial history of psoriasis of the child.

In fact, approximately 30% of children with psoriasis have a familial history of psoriasis with an affected first-degree relative and it has been estimated that if one parent is affected by psoriasis, the child has an estimated risk to develop disease of about 25%, while if the two parents are affected, the child has an estimated risk of 60–70% [2, 4–9].

Collecting medical history data of the child, it should be also investigated and considered the potential trigger factors which could be related to the onset of psoriasis.

A common trigger factor of psoriasis in the pediatric age which should be always investigated is related to pharyngeal and perianal infections by groups A, C, and G b-hemolytic streptococci. These infections are commonly linked to the onset and exacerbation of guttate psoriasis and a swab of the involved site should be taken for culture in case of suspected streptococcal infection [5–9, 13–21].

Other environmental trigger factors which could be related to the psoriasis' onset and which should be investigated include emotional or physical stress, skin trauma or local skin irritation, smoking (more important in the teenager population), and drugs (such as sodium valproate, non-steroidal anti-inflammatory, some mental health drugs, b-blockers, and anti-malarial drugs) [13–21].

A complete physical examination of the child, in the case of a suspected diagnosis of psoriasis, is also recommended; all the skin of body, nails, and also mucosa should be observed.

Fissured and geographic tongue (also defined as "*benign migratory glossitis*") are common reported oral lesions; the incidence of geographic tongue increases as the severity of psoriasis increases in adults, with several cases reported also in children with plaque psoriasis [22–24].

Clinical severity assessment of psoriasis can be performed using several tools in order to monitor the efficacy of the treatments.

5.1   Clinical Severity Assessment

Many tools and scores are available in children in order to assess the severity of pediatric psoriasis (Table 5.1).

5.1.1   Psoriasis Area Severity Index (PASI)

Psoriasis Area Severity Index (PASI) score is considered the gold standard to assess the severity of psoriasis and is usually used in clinical trials in adults and in children.

PASI score takes into account several clinical parameters of skin lesions, assigned by an evaluator (a dermatologist or a trained physician): erythema, thickness, scaliness, and the percentage of affected area considering four body section (head and neck, trunk, upper limbs and lower limbs).

PASI score ranges from 0 to 72 and its use is validated in older children and adults. Psoriasis is considered severe when the PASI score is ≥10.

A 75% reduction in the PASI score (PASI 75) is the current benchmark for most clinical trials in psoriasis and the criterion for efficacy of new psoriasis treatments.

PASI score tries to give an objective measurement of the severity of psoriasis, although it has significant limitations because it does not consider other, not less important, parameters related to the disease (such as pruritus or the impact on quality of life of patient) [2, 5–11].

5.1.2   Investigator Global Assessment (IGA)

The Investigator Global Assessment (IGA) score is based on a point-in-time assessment.

It is a relatively simple and easy score with a good correlation with PASI score. It has high clinical construct validity and a great test–retest reliability, with a

Table 5.1 Tools and scores commonly used to assess the severity of psoriasis and quality of life in children

Score	Parameters	Range	Severity stratification
Psoriasis Area Severity Index (PASI)	• Erythema; • Induration; • Scaling; • Percentage of involved surface area in four specific section: head, neck, trunk, upper limbs, lower limbs.	0–72	• PASI <10: mild psoriasis • PASI ≥10: moderate-to-severe psoriasis
Body Surface Area (BSA)	• Percentage of skin body area affected by psoriasis; • 1% is considered corresponding to the palm, fingers, and thumb area of patient.	0–100%	• BSA <3%: mild psoriasis • BSA 3–10%: moderate psoriasis • BSA >10%: severe psoriasis
Investigator Global Assessment (IGA)	Over the entire body area: • Hyperpigmentation • Thickening • Coloration	0–4	• 0: clear (e.g., no signs of psoriasis, some post-inflammatory hyperpigmentation) • 1: almost clear (e.g., no thickening, normal or pink coloration) • 2: mild (e.g., mild thickening, pink to light red coloration) • 3: moderate (e.g., moderate thickening, dull to bright red) • 4: severe (e.g., severe thickening, bright to deep red)
Physician Global Assessment (PGA)	Over the entire body area: • Erythema • Thickness • Scaliness	0–4	• 0: clear • 1: almost clear • 2: mild • 3: moderate • 4: severe
Children's Dermatology Life Quality Index (CDLQI)	Questionnaire with 10 questions investigating: • Symptoms • Feelings • Leisure • School activities • Personal and familiar relationships • Quality of sleep • Impact on quality of life due to the treatment	0–30	• 0–1: no effect on child's life • 2–6: small effect • 7–12: moderate effect • 13–18: very large effect • 19–30: extremely large effect

moderate agreement among multiple investigators. IGA score is commonly used by investigator in clinical trials to evaluate the severity of psoriasis.

However, IGA score should be used in association with other scores, as it is not able to measure the extent of the diseases and has a low sensitivity to small changes in psoriasis' severity [10–14].

5.1.3   Physician Global Assessment (PGA)

The Physician Global Assessment (PGA) score and affected Body Surface Area (BSA) score could be considered an alternative for PASI.

The PGA score considers three clinical parameters of psoriatic lesions (degree of erythema, thickness, and scaliness) over the entire body, resulting in a value ranging from 0 (clear) to 4 (severe).

The PGA is more subjective than PASI (in which there is no attempt to quantify the individual elements of plaque morphology) or than Body Surface Area score [25, 26].

5.1.4   Body Surface Area (BSA)

Another simple score is the Body Surface Area (BSA) score, which considers the percentage of skin body area affected by psoriasis, where 1% corresponds to the palm, fingers, and thumb area of each patient. Psoriasis is considered mild when skin lesions cover less than 3% of total body area, moderate skin lesions cover less than 3–10% of total body area and severe when over 10% of total body area is affected [25].

5.1.5   Nail Psoriasis Severity Index (NAPSI), Psoriasis Nail Severity Score (PNSS)

Some simple tools have been developed as objective and reproducible instruments in order to evaluate the severity of psoriasis in case of nail involvement, helping to estimate the nail involvement and to standardize the treatment outcome assessment.

These scores are the Nail Psoriasis Severity Index (NAPSI) and the Psoriasis Nail Severity Score (PNSS).

The NAPSI score evaluates the psoriatic changes of the nails considering the nail divided with imaginary horizontal and longitudinal lines into quadrants. For each nail the NAPSI score can amount to 8 points, considering a score for bad nail lesions (0–4 points) and a score for nail matrices (0–4 points) depending on the presence of any of the typical clinical features in that quadrant (pitting, red spots, leukonychia, onycholysis, nail plate crumbling, dyschromia, subungual hyperkeratosis, and splinter hemorrhages) [27, 28].

The Psoriasis Nail Severity Score (PNSS) assigns one point for the presence of each clinical change among these: pitting, subungual hyperkeratosis, onycholysis, and advanced deformation of both nail ends. The maximum score is 4 for a nail [27, 28].

5.2 Assessment of Comorbidities

Psoriasis in adults is associated with several systemic diseases, and more and more evidence are available about the association of the same comorbidities with pediatric psoriasis. Cardiovascular and metabolic diseases are the principal systemic comorbidities of psoriasis both in adults and children. The relatively recent concept of the "psoriatic march" could explain the association between these comorbidities and psoriasis, as the systemic and chronic inflammation in psoriasis may cause insulin resistance, triggering endothelial cell dysfunction and leading to atherosclerosis and increasing the risk of myocardial infarction and stroke. On the other hand, in over-weight and obese patients with psoriasis the systemic inflammation is further increased as the adipose tissue acts as an endocrine tissue, releasing pro-inflammatory cytokines [29–33].

A special attention should be given to the screening and monitoring the parameters related to some metabolic and cardiovascular comorbidities in children with psoriasis.

Hypertension, hyperlipidemia, over-weight/obesity, diabetes mellitus, and metabolic syndrome have recently been noted associated with psoriasis also in children and adolescents.

5.2.1 Over-Weight, Obesity, and Central Obesity

Children with psoriasis are at higher risk of being over-weight or obese.

The calculation of Body Mass Index (BMI) is a simple tool useful to determine the status of normal-, over-weight, or obesity of the child.

BMI corresponds to weight in kilograms divided by height in meters squared; the child is over-weight when BMI is ≥85th percentile to <95th percentile for age and sex, and obese when BMI is ≥ 95th percentile.

Central obesity (also known as "abdominal obesity") refers to the abdominal fat mass and it is a condition related to an excessive of visceral fat around the stomach.

Central obesity has been found strongly related to cardiovascular and metabolic diseases, including an altered lipid profile, high blood pressure, and impaired glucose tolerance and insulin sensitivity that have been reported to originate early in childhood.

Several studies found a correlation between psoriasis and central obesity in children with psoriasis, reporting that children with psoriasis have a higher risk to have central obesity compared to psoriasis-free control subjects [7, 13, 14, 29–33].

Therefore, central obesity represents a relevant link between psoriasis and the several associated metabolic and cardiovascular diseases.

A common tool that could be used in children with psoriasis in order to assess and to determine central obesity is the Waist to Height Ratio (WHtR). WHtR is an important parameter considered strictly related to the metabolic condition and to the risk of developing metabolic diseases; it was found to be higher in patients with moderate to severe psoriasis, suggesting an increased risk for metabolic and cardiovascular disease.

Central obesity seems to be associated with psoriasis also in normal-weight children, suggesting that this condition is correlated to psoriasis independently from the weight of patient.

There is also an association between weight and severity of psoriasis, as weight seems increasing with psoriasis severity, with some evidence showing that adiposity could precede psoriatic lesions by 2 years in a majority of children with psoriasis.

In children with psoriasis, a screening for over-weight and obesity should be performed yearly using BMI percentile, starting at 2 years of age [34–36].

In children with over-weight, obesity or central obesity, physicians should discuss with patients and families the importance of early performing lifestyle changes in order to reduce any additional risk, also considering that psoriasis alone has been found to be an independent risk factor for cardiovascular and metabolic diseases in adulthood.

5.2.2   Hypertension, Hyperlipidemia, and Diabetes Mellitus

An association of higher blood pressure in children with psoriasis independently of weight has been reported [37].

Screen for hypertension in children with psoriasis should be performed yearly in children older than 3 years old, using age, sex, and height reference charts [34–36].

Children with psoriasis seem also report elevated plasma lipids compared to healthy controls and also independently of BMI; these data suggest that psoriasis itself could lead to metabolic alterations [7, 13, 14, 30].

Hyperlipidemia represents a relevant metabolic alteration that could arise early in childhood and an universal lipid screening during the following 2 age ranges (9–11 years old and 17–21 years old) is recommended in children and adolescents with psoriasis [34–36].

Children with psoriasis seem also at higher risk to develop diabetes mellitus and metabolic syndrome compared to healthy psoriasis-free children. It is recommended to screen using fasting serume glucose, every 3 years, starting at age 10 years or at the onset of puberty in over-weight and obese children with psoriasis [34–36].

5.2.3   Arthritis

Psoriatic arthritis is a form of arthritis or joint inflammation that affects both skin and joints.

Psoriatic arthritis causes joint pain and painful swelling, often affecting finger and toe joints; however, it can also affect wrists, ankles, knees, and the lower back.

This condition is most common in adults ages 30 to 50 years old, but it can start in childhood.

Juvenile psoriatic arthritis is another manifestation of psoriasis in children [5–7].

The peak of onset in childhood is between ages 9 and 12, and the skin psoriasis often precedes psoriatic arthritis [7].

Psoriatic arthritis could be very destructive and debilitating and its early identification, diagnosis, and intervention in childhood are a priority, helping to ease pain and prevent joint damage from getting worse.

Clinical characteristics of psoriatic arthritis during the first peak (2–3 years of age) are similar to those of juvenile idiopathic arthritis, showing a female predisposition, antinuclear antibody positivity, and oligoarthritis or polyarthritis with a common small joint involvement. During the second peak (10–12 years of age), the characteristics seem to be more similar to spondyloarthritis: male predisposition, enthesitis, axial disease, and HLA-B27 positivity [34, 38, 39].

In pediatric psoriatic arthritis, the dactylitis (inflammation of an entire digit) is a common finding. Most of children with psoriatic arthritis develop arthritis 2–3 years prior to the onset of skin lesions, whereas adult patients tend to develop skin manifestations of psoriasis before arthritis symptoms.

Children with psoriasis should be carefully screened for the development of arthritis by a directed review of symptoms and physical examination [34–36].

Although several arthritis screening tools have been created for adult patients with psoriasis, none is actually validated in children.

Screening questions should be asked to the child and his parents in order to evaluate limp and stiffness, and investigating joint pain (knees, ankles, wrists) particularly in the morning.

Furthermore, physicians should be considered that there is a strong association between nail psoriasis involvement and the risk of psoriatic arthritis [34–39].

The prevalence of nail involvement among patients with psoriatic arthritis is as high as 70%. In particular, nail involvement may precede arthritis or may be considered as a predictor of future psoriatic joint damage. A possible explanation for this association could be the close anatomical link between the nail unit and the distal interphalangeal joint. Inflammation of the extensor tendon enthesis, that are the attachment points of ligaments, tendons, and joint capsules to bone, can extend to the nail unit and result in psoriatic nail alterations [28].

Therefore, children with nail involvement should be investigated for the presence of psoriatic arthritis [34–36].

A simple tool developed as an objective and reproducible instrument, which helps to estimate the nail involvement and therefore to standardize the treatment outcome assessments, is the Nail Psoriasis Severity Index (NAPSI).

5.2.4   Psychiatric Comorbidities

While adults with psoriasis have increased risk of depression and other psychiatric disorders, limited data are available about the incidence of psychiatric comorbidities among pediatric patients with psoriasis.

Some studies were conducted in Europe and in USA, finding that children with psoriasis have higher risk for psychiatric diseases (such as depression, anxiety, and bipolar disease) compared with children without. Furthermore, these studies suggested that children with psoriasis may be at high risk for psychiatric treatment of psychiatric disorders [5, 34, 36, 38–40].

The association between psoriasis and psychiatric diseases could be related to several factors; in fact, psoriasis often causes a social stigmatization since pediatric age, resulting in behavioral changes. On the other hand, depression could lead to increased risk behavior.

Considering the multidimensional impact of psoriasis on the life of children and adolescents, it should be also considered that psoriasis often confers a significant psychosocial disease burden, with an increased risk of several psychiatric disorders and treatment for psychiatric diseases, also in children. Therefore, these comorbidities should be early investigated and recognized in childhood psoriasis, allowing for an early treatment [5, 34, 36, 38–40].

5.2.5   Gastrointestinal Diseases

Adult patients with psoriasis seem to be at higher risk to develop inflammatory bowel diseases (both Crohn disease and ulcerative colitis) and celiac disease.

In children with psoriasis showing decreased growth rate, unexplained weight loss or symptoms consistent with inflammatory bowel disease or celiac disease (abdominal pain, nausea, vomiting, diarrhea), a formal gastrointestinal evaluation is recommended [5, 34, 36, 38, 39].

5.3   Assessment of the Quality of Life

Psoriasis in children has a great impact on the quality of life of patients and this aspect should be monitored like the clinical severity of disease. A simple tool that is commonly used to assess the quality of life related to chronic skin dermatoses in children is the Children's Dermatology Life Quality Index (CDLQI) score. CDLQI score is calculated through a questionnaire, specifically structured to investigate the quality of life in pediatric age.

The questionnaire consists of 10 multiple choice questions with a unique possible answer, exploring several areas of children's life (such as symptoms due to disease, personal sensations, school and sport activities, interpersonal and familiar relationships, and quality of sleep). Total CDLQI score derives from the scores of the 10 question items, ranging from 0 (no impact on quality of life) to 19–30 (extremely large impact on quality of life) [41–43].

It is demonstrated that the severity of impact on quality of life due to psoriasis in children is related, not only to the severity of disease, but also to the presence of skin lesions in visible areas (such as face, hands), underlying the psychological impact that the disease could have, especially in adolescents [44].

Therefore, the evaluation of severity of childhood psoriasis should be multidimensional, considering several tools assessing the different aspects of the disease, such as the impact on the quality of life which could be significantly impaired even with minimal involved body surface area [44–46].

As many inflammatory chronic skin diseases, psoriasis is known to have a great impact on the lives, not only of the patients, but also of their families. Family Dermatology Life Quality Index (FDLQI) is a validate dermatology-specific instrument useful to evaluate and quantify the impact on the quality of life of family member of patients with skin diseases [47].

Family members play a central role in the care of such patients, especially in children with inflammatory chronic skin diseases; family impact data are potentially important components of the measurement of the overall burden of skin disease which should be evaluated and considered. FDLQI is a simple and user-friendly tool useful for clinical use, consisting of 10 multiple choice questions addressed to family members of the patient, with a unique possible answer and with a total score ranging from 0 to 30 [47].

References

1. Megna M, Napolitano M, Balato A, et al. Psoriasis in children: a review. Curr Pediatr Rev. 2015;11(1):10–26.
2. Mahé E. Childhood psoriasis. Eur J Dermatol. 2016;26(6):537–48.
3. Dhar S, Banerjee R, Agrawal N, et al. Psoriasis in children: an insight. Indian J Dermatol. 2011;56(3):262–5.
4. Relvas M, Torres T. Pediatric psoriasis. Am J Clin Dermatol. 2017;18(6):797–811.
5. Tolliver S, Pepper AN, Pothiawala S, Silverberg NB. Pediatric psoriasis. In: Weinberg JM, Lebwohl M, editors. Advances in psoriasis. Cham: Springer; 2021.
6. Eichenfield LF, Paller AS, Tom WL, et al. Pediatric psoriasis: evolving perspectives. Pediatr Dermatol. 2018 Mar;35(2):170–81.
7. Bronckers IM, Paller AS, van Geel MJ, van de Kerkhof PC, Seyger MM. Psoriasis in children and adolescents: diagnosis. Management and comorbidities. Paediatr Drugs. 2015;17(5):373–84.
8. Pinson R, Sotoodian B, Fiorillo L. Psoriasis in children. Psoriasis (Auckl). 2016;6:121–9.
9. Seyhan M, Coskun BK, Saglam H, et al. Psoriasis in childhood and adolescence: evaluation of demographic and clinical features. Pediatr Int. 2006;48:525–30.
10. Boehncke WH, Schon MP. Psoriasis. Lancet. 2015;386(9997):983–94.
11. Van de Kerkhof PCM, Schalkwijk J. Psoriasis. In: Bolognia JL, Jorizzo JL, Rapini RP, editors. Dermatology. 2nd ed. Philadelphia: Mosby Elsevier; 2008.
12. Silverberg NB. Update on pediatric psoriasis, part 1: clinical features and demographics. Cutis. 2010;86(3):118–24.
13. Tollefson MM. Diagnosis and management of psoriasis in children. Pediatr Clin N Am. 2014;61(2):261–77.
14. Cordoro KM. Management of childhood psoriasis. Adv Dermatol. 2008;28:125–69.
15. Shah KN. Diagnosis and treatment of pediatric psoriasis: current and future. Am J Clin Dermatol. 2013;14(3):195–213.
16. Murphy M, Kerr P, Grant-Kels JM. The histopathologic spectrum of psoriasis. Clin Dermatol. 2007;25(6):524–8.
17. Gupta MA, Gupta AK, Watteel GN. Cigarette smoking in men may be a risk factor for increased severity of psoriasis of the extremities. Br J Dermatol. 1996;135(5):859–60.
18. Ozden MG, Tekin NS, Gurer MA, et al. Environmental risk factors in pediatric psoriasis: a multicenter case–control study. Pediatr Dermatol. 2011;28(3):306–12.

19. Basavaraj KH, Ashok NM, Rashmi R, Praveen TK. The role of drugs in the induction and/or exacerbation of psoriasis. Int J Dermatol. 2010;49(12):1351–61.
20. Gudjonsson JE, Thorarinsson AM, Sigurgeirsson B, et al. Streptococcal throat infections and exacerbation of chronic plaque psoriasis: a prospective study. Br J Dermatol. 2003;149(3):530–4.
21. Gul Mert G, Incecik F, Gunasti S, et al. Psoriasiform drug eruption associated with sodium valproate. Case Rep Pediatr. 2013;2013:823469.
22. Yesudian PD, Chalmers RJ, Warren RB, Griffiths CE. In search of oral psoriasis. Arch Dermatol Res. 2012;304(1):1–5.
23. Daneshpazhooh M, Moslehi H, Akhyani M, EtesamiM. Tongue lesions in psoriasis: a controlled study. BMC Dermatol 2004;4(1):16.
24. Cambiaghi S, Colonna C, Cavalli R. Geographic tongue in two children with nonpustular psoriasis. Pediatr Dermatol. 2005;22(1):83–5.
25. Hani AF, Prakasa E, Nugroho H, et al. Body surface area measurement and soft clustering for PASI area assessment. Conf Proc IEEE Eng Med Biol Soc. 2012;2012:4398–401.
26. Walsh JA, McFadden M, Woodcock J, et al. Product of the physician global assessment and body surface area: a simple static measure of psoriasis severity in a longitudinal cohort. J Am Acad Dermatol. 2013;69(6):931–7.
27. Oram Y, Akkaya AD. Treatment of nail psoriasis: common concepts and new trends. Dermatol Res Pract. 2013;2013:180496.
28. Sobolewski P, Walecka I, Dopytalska K. Nail involvement in psoriatic arthritis. Reumatologia. 2017;55(3):131–5.
29. Caroppo F, Belloni FA. Psoriasis and comorbidities in children. Arch Pediatr. 2019 May;26(4):247.
30. Busch AL, Landau JM, Moody MN, Goldberg LH. Pediatric psoriasis. Skin Ther Lett. 2012;17(1):5–7.
31. Mortz CG, Brockow K, Bindslev-Jensen C, Broesby-Olsen S. It looks like childhood eczema but is it? Clin Exp Allergy. 2019;49(6):744–53.
32. Guidolin L, Borin M, Fontana E, Caroppo F, Piaserico S, Fortina AB. Central obesity in children with psoriasis. Acta Derm Venereol. 2018;98(2):282–3.
33. Caroppo F, Galderisi A, Ventura L, Belloni FA. Metabolic syndrome and insulin resistance in pre-pubertal children with psoriasis. Eur J Pediatr. 2021;180(6):1739–45.
34. Osier E, Wang AS, Tollefson MM, et al. Pediatric psoriasis comorbidity screening guidelines. JAMA Dermatol. 2017;153(7):698–704.
35. Stahle M, Atakan N, Boehncke WH, et al. Juvenile psoriasis and its clinical management: a European expert group consensus. J Dtsch Dermatol Ges. 2010;8(10):812–8.
36. Paller AS, Schenfeld J, Accortt NA, Kricorian G. A retrospective cohort study to evaluate the development of comorbidities, including psychiatric comorbidities, among a pediatric psoriasis population. Pediatr Dermatol. 2019;36(3):290–7.
37. Caroppo F, Ventura L, Belloni FA. High blood pressure in normal-weight children with psoriasis. Acta Derm Venereol. 2019;99(3):329–30.
38. Kang BY, O'Haver J, Andrews ID. Pediatric psoriasis comorbidities: screening recommendations for the primary care provider. J Pediatr Health Care. 2021;35(3):337–50.
39. Edson-Heredia E, Anderson S, Guo J, et al. Real-world claims analyses of comorbidity burden. Treatment pattern: healthcare resource utilization, and costs in pediatric psoriasis. Adv Ther. 2021;38(7):3948–61.
40. Todberg T, Egeberg A, Jensen P, Gislason G, Skov L. Psychiatric comorbidities in children and adolescents with psoriasis: a population-based cohort study. Br J Dermatol. 2017;177(2):551–3.
41. Lewis-Jones MS, Ay F. The Children's Dermatology Life Quality Index (CDLQI): initial validation and practical use. Br J Dermatol. 1995;132:942–9.
42. Cardiff University Department of Dermatology and Wound Healing. Children's Dermatology Life Quality Index CDLQI: different language versions. Available at: http://www.dermatology.org.uk/quality/cdlqi/quality-cdlqilanguages.html

43. Waters A, Sandhu D, Beattie P, Ezughah F, Lewis-Jones S. Severity stratification of Children's Dermatology Life Quality Index (CDLQI) scores. Br J Dermatol. 2010;163:121.
44. Caroppo F, Zacchino M, Milazzo E, Fontana E, Nobile F, Marogna C, Ventura L, Belloni FA. Quality of life in children with psoriasis: results from a monocentric study. G Ital Dermatol Venereol. 2019;156(3):374–7.
45. Randa H, Todberg T, Skov L, Larsen LS, Zachariae R. Health related quality of life in children and adolescents with psoriasis: a systematic review and meta-analysis. Acta Derm Venereol. 2017;97(5):555–63.
46. De Jager ME, De Jong EM, Evers AW, Van De Kerkhof PC, Seyger MM. The burden of childhood psoriasis. Pediatr Dermatol. 2011;28:736–7.
47. Basra MK, Sue-Ho R, Finlay AY. The Family Dermatology Life Quality Index: measuring the secondary impact of skin disease. Br J Dermatol. 2007;156(3):528–38.

Differential Diagnosis

6

Although the principal clinical subtypes of psoriasis in children are the same of psoriasis in adults, skin lesions may differ about distribution and morphology in pediatric age. Lesions of psoriasis in children are in fact generally thinner, smaller, and less scaly and the involvement of some body areas (such as the scalp, face, and anogenital regions) is more common in children than in the adults [1–5].

Therefore, the diagnosis of psoriasis in children and adolescents may be more challenging when compared to the well-delineated features of psoriasis in adults, also considering that formal diagnostic criteria for psoriasis do not exist, the diagnosis is primarily based on clinical manifestations and on anamnestic findings and that skin biopsy is rarely performed in pediatric age.

The differential diagnoses of psoriasis can greatly vary depending on the clinical subtypes of disease and locations of the skin lesions (Table 6.1)

Particular attention should be paid to the morphology of cutaneous lesions, the involved body areas, familial history of psoriasis, nail and mucosal aspects, and the possible presence of atopic signs.

Therefore, a correct diagnosis of psoriasis also depends on the specific experience, clinical skills, and on the knowledge of the possible differential diagnosis of psoriasis in children by the physicians.

In fact, childhood psoriasis could be misdiagnosed as several inflammatory skin conditions in children, such as atopic dermatitis, irritant or allergic contact dermatitis, nummular eczema, dyshidrotic eczema, pityriasis rosea, lichen planus, seborrheic dermatitis, and pityriasis rubra pilaris [3–7].

Psoriasis may also mimic some skin infectious conditions, such as tinea infections, candida infections, blistering dactylitis, and onychomycosis [4–8].

Other possible differential diagnosis which should be considered, especially in case of severe psoriasis with an extensive involvement of skin body area, include cutaneous T-cell lymphoma and staphylococcal scalded skin syndrome.

The differential diagnoses of childhood psoriasis can be summarized depending on the suspected clinical subtype of psoriasis (Table 6.1)

© The Author(s), under exclusive license to Springer Nature
Switzerland AG 2022
A. Belloni Fortina, F. Caroppo, *Pediatric Psoriasis*,
https://doi.org/10.1007/978-3-030-90712-9_6

Table 6.1 Differential diagnoses of pediatric psoriasis

Clinical subtype of psoriasis	Differential diagnoses
Guttate psoriasis	• Pityriasis lichenoides chronica • Pityriasis rosea (typical evolution with bimodal course: "herald patch" followed, 7–14 days after, by many smaller but similar lesions on the trunk, and clinical appearance) • Secondary syphilis (involvement of palmoplantar region, history of unsafe sexual intercourse, positive serology) • Lichen ruber planus (well-defined areas of purple-colored, itchy, flat-topped papules with interspersed lacy white lines -Wickham's striae, the distribution of the lesions, frequent severe itching) • Pityriasis rubra pilaris (yellowish, salmon-like lesions with sparing islands on the trunk, distribution of the lesions and age of onset) • Tinea corporis (evolution of the lesions, extension, mycological examination) • Nummular dermatitis
Inverse psoriasis	• Irritant/allergic contact dermatitis (correlation between the rash and the culprit, patch test positive in case of allergic contact dermatitis) • Intertrigo (borders are not well edged) • Candidiasis (peripheral pustules, positive mycological examination) • Darier's/Hailey-Hailey disease • Erythrasma
Plaque psoriasis/ scalp psoriasis	• Atopic dermatitis (family history for atopy, oozing lesions, cheilitis, infra-auricular fissure, itching, localization, Dennie-Morgan folds and evolution of the lesions with age) • Atopic dermatitis/psoriasis overlap • Pityriasis rubra pilaris (yellowish, salmon-like lesions with sparing islands on the trunk, distribution of the lesions and age of onset) • Seborrheic dermatitis (scaly, greasy patches; different histological features) • Tinea capitis (patchy alopecia, slowly enlarging with fine scales; mycological examination) • Tinea corporis (evolution of the lesions, extension, mycological examination) • Nummular eczema (exudative and itchy lesions)
Nail psoriasis	• Onychomycosis (absent pitting, positive mycological examination) • Lichen ruber planus (grooved and ridged nail plates, possible pterygium and 20-nail dystrophy) • Trauma
Follicular psoriasis	• Lichen ruber planus (well-defined areas of purple-colored, itchy, flat-topped papules with interspersed lacy white lines -Wickham's striae, the distribution of the lesions, frequent severe itching) • Pityriasis rubra pilaris (yellowish, salmon-like lesions with sparing islands on the trunk, distribution of the lesions and age of onset) • Lichen spinulosus (most commonly single lesions—patches of stippled and spiny papules centered on hair follicles, like a "nutmeg grater," symmetrically involving elbows, knees, trunk, buttocks) • Follicular eczema

(continued)

Table 6.1 (continued)

Clinical subtype of psoriasis	Differential diagnoses
Erythrodermic psoriasis	• Pityriasis rubra pilaris (yellowish, salmon-like lesions with sparing islands on the trunk, distribution of the lesions and age of onset) • Atopic dermatitis (family history for atopy, oozing lesions, cheilitis, infra-auricular fissure, itching, localization, Dennie-Morgan folds and evolution of the lesions with age) • Mycosis fungoides • Congenital nonbullous ichthyosiform • Lichen ruber planus
Pustular psoriasis	• SSSS (Staphylococcal scalded skin syndrome) • Blistering distal dactylitis • Acute generalized exanthematous pustulosis • Sweet syndrome

6.1   Guttate Psoriasis

Guttate psoriasis (or "drop-like" psoriasis) is a clinical subtype of psoriasis which is more common in children and adolescents than in adults and is clinically characterized by a diffuse, widespread acute eruption with small (usually less than 1 cm), dot-shaped, red-to-salmon-colored plaques with fine desquamation.

Among the different clinical subtypes of psoriasis, guttate psoriasis is the form most commonly related to a previous infection as principal recognized trigger factor. In particular, guttate psoriasis is often preceded by a group A beta hemolytic streptococcus infection of the upper respiratory tract in the most of cases and, less frequently, of other body areas (such as perianal or vulvar regions) [1, 2, 3, 5, 7–12].

The principal differential diagnoses of guttate psoriasis include several inflammatory skin conditions and dermatoses, such as pityriasis lichenoides chronica, pityriasis rosea, pityriasis rubra pilaris, and lichen ruber planus.

Pityriasis lichenoides chronica is a relatively rare idiopathic dermatosis characterized by moderate-to-severe recurrent eruptions of small scaly red-brownish or erythematous papules which evolve into blisters and crusted red-brown spots, generally involving trunk, upper, and lower limbs and often hesitating in hypopigmented macules.

Pityriasis rosea commonly has its onset on the trunk with oval scaly papules and plaques organized along skin tension lines in a typical "Christmas tree" pattern, with the presence of a herald patch and generally a spontaneous resolution in few months.

In skin lesions of pityriasis lichenoides chronica and pityriasis rosea, Auspitz sign when the scale is lifted off is absent.

Pityriasis rubra pilaris is a dermatosis characterized by reddish-orange colored scaling papules and patches with well-defined border involving extensive body areas or specific body regions such as knees and elbows. Pityriasis rubra pilaris is clinically distinguished from plaque psoriasis by the presence of keratotic follicular papules, the classic areas of sparing on the trunk, and red-orange palmoplantar keratoderma.

Lichen ruber planus is a benign dermatosis, rarely observed in children, which can mimic guttate or plaque psoriasis. Lichen ruber planus is characterized by purple-to-violaceus, pruritic skin papules generally involving the flexor surfaces of the wrists and ankles.

When the lesions are more limited number or are anular, tinea corporis is another possible differential diagnosis of guttate psoriasis or plaque psoriasis [12–16].

In doubtful cases, the characteristic psoriatic lesions in particular body areas (such as scalp, retroauricular regions, periumbilical or genital regions) and familial history of psoriasis should be always investigated.

6.2   Inverse Psoriasis

Inverse psoriasis is more common in children than in adults, affecting most frequently infants and young children.

The most affected areas of inverse psoriasis are the flexural and intertriginous regions, including axillae, retro-auricular regions, inguinal folds, and genital or perianal areas. In infants the most frequent clinical type of psoriasis is a specific form of inverse psoriasis related to the involvement of diaper area, delineating the specific clinical subtype of "napkin psoriasis."

The most common differential diagnosis of diaper psoriasis in infants is the irritant or allergic contact dermatitis. Diaper psoriasis can be differentiated from irritant or allergic napkin dermatitis, investigating the involvement of the entire fold areas, which is typical of napkin psoriasis and is usually absent in irritant napkin dermatitis [1–5, 9–12].

Inverse psoriasis can also be a common cause of intertrigo and intertrigo is a possible differential diagnosis of inverse psoriasis which should be considered, especially in infants.

Other possible etiologies of skin infections in inverse psoriasis include tinea corporis and cutaneous candidiasis. Candidiasis usually presents with a beefy red color and satellite pustules.

Suspecting a cutaneous infection in skin lesions of inverse psoriasis, it is recommended to use topical anti-infective drugs or to require specific skin cultures.

The frequency of involvement of anogenital regions in children with inverse psoriasis generally decreases with increasing age of the child and inverse psoriasis later tends to present in other body areas or with more typical lesions of the classic plaque-type psoriasis.

6.3   Plaque-Type and Scalp Psoriasis

Plaque-type psoriasis and scalp psoriasis are common clinical types of psoriasis in children and adolescents.

The prevalence of pediatric plaque-type and scalp psoriasis increases with age, reaching more than 70% in adolescents.

Plaque-type psoriasis in children can involve some typical body areas (such as the elbows, knees, and scalp), but some locations are more frequent in childhood, such as anogenital and facial areas [1–5].

The typical skin lesions of plaque-type psoriasis are generally monomorphic, well demarcated, red plaques, covered by gray lamellar scales.

In younger children, the clinical aspect may be atypical, with smaller, more pink, less scaly and less demarcated lesions, often resembling an atopic dermatitis. In fact, the main differential diagnosis of plaque-type psoriasis in younger children can be considered an eczema-psoriasis overlap (also called "*eczemoriasis*") [5, 6].

The most common differential diagnoses of plaque-type psoriasis in children also include nummular dermatitis, tinea corporis, and pityriasis rubra pilaris.

Pityriasis rubra pilaris may be clinically distinguished from plaque-type psoriasis by the presence of keratotic follicular papules and the typical sparing islands of the trunk.

Scalp psoriasis is another common clinical type of psoriasis in children and adolescents; scalp psoriasis can show an involvement only of scalp or also of other body areas with the typical skin lesions of plaque-type psoriasis.

A common differential diagnosis of scalp psoriasis is seborrheic dermatitis, a common dermatosis of adolescents. Scalp psoriasis could be distinguished from seborrheic dermatitis as scalp psoriasis is characterized by asymmetrical, sharply demarcated skin lesions showing a white-silver scaling, often itching. The scales in psoriatic lesions are generally dry, shiny, and whitish, while those of seborrheic dermatitis are more yellowish and greasy.

Another common differential diagnosis of scalp psoriasis, especially in children, is tinea capitis; tinea capitis is generally characterized by broken-off stumps of hair, also often with crusts and pustules on the scalp [3, 5, 6, 13–17].

6.4   Nail Psoriasis

Nail psoriasis is less common in children than in adults, but often this finding could be underdiagnosed or not reported in children affected by other clinical type of psoriasis.

Clinical characteristics of nail psoriasis are pitting, discoloration of the nail plate with brownish-yellowish patches, onycholysis, onychodystrophy, and subungual hyperkeratosis. The involved nails are generally more than one in fingers and toes [1–7, 17].

Some clinical findings of nail psoriasis can overlap with other nail conditions (such as onychomycosis and trauma); the differential diagnoses should consider the involvement of one or more nails, familial history of psoriasis and the evidence of psoriatic skin lesions in other body areas.

References

1. Megna M, Napolitano M, Balato A, et al. Psoriasis in children: a review. Curr Pediatr Rev. 2015;11(1):10–26.
2. Relvas M, Torres T. Pediatric psoriasis. Am J Clin Dermatol. 2017;18(6):797–811.
3. Sarkar S, Dhar S, Raychaudhuri SP. Childhood psoriasis: disease spectrum, comorbidities, and challenges. Indian J Paediatr Dermatol. 2019;20:191–8.
4. Mahé E. Childhood psoriasis. Eur J Dermatol. 2016;26(6):537–48.
5. Forward E, Lee G, Fischer G. Shades of grey: what is paediatric psoriasiform dermatitis and what does it have in common with childhood psoriasis? Clin Exp Dermatol. 2021;46(1):65–73.
6. Mortz CG, Brockow K, Bindslev-Jensen C, Broesby-Olsen S. It looks like childhood eczema but is it? Clin Exp Allergy. 2019;49(6):744–53.
7. Eichenfield LF, Paller AS, Tom WL, et al. Pediatric psoriasis: evolving perspectives. Pediatr Dermatol. 2018;35(2):170–81.
8. Shah KN. Diagnosis and treatment of pediatric psoriasis: current and future. Am J Clin Dermatol. 2013;14(3):195–213.
9. Mahé E, Gnossike P, Sigal ML. Childhood psoriasis. Arch Pediatr. 2014;21(7):778–86.
10. Balato N, Di Costanzo L, Balato A. Differential diagnosis of psoriasis. J Rheumatol Suppl. 2009;83:24–5.
11. Naldi L, Gambini D. The clinical spectrum of psoriasis. Clin Dermatol. 2007;25(6):510–8.
12. Barisic-Drusko V, Rucevic I. Psoriasis in childhood. Coll Anthropol. 2004;1:211–85.
13. Silverberg NB. Update on pediatric psoriasis, part 1: clinical features and demographics. Cutis. 2010;86(3):118–24.
14. Mercy K, Kwasny M, Cordoro KM, et al. Clinical manifestations of pediatric psoriasis: results of a multicenter study in the United States. Pediatr Dermatol. 2013;30(4):424–8.
15. Tollefson MM. Diagnosis and management of psoriasis in children. Pediatr Clin N Am. 2014;61(2):261–77.
16. Bronckers IM, Paller AS, van Geel MJ, van de Kerkhof PC, Seyger MM. Psoriasis in children and adolescents: diagnosis, management and comorbidities. Paediatr Drugs. 2015;17(5):373–84.
17. Tolliver S, Pepper AN, Pothiawala S, Silverberg NB. Pediatric psoriasis. In: Weinberg JM, Lebwohl M, editors. Advances in psoriasis. Cham: Springer; 2021.

Treatment

7

The treatment and management of psoriasis can be very challenging, especially in children, requiring a careful compliance to specific and several therapies.

Particular attention should be paid, not only to find the best treatment for the clinical type and the severity of psoriasis, but also to provide an educational therapy to the child and to the parents, explaining them that the pathogenesis of psoriasis is based on genetic and immunological factors, that the disease is chronic with an alternation of remissions and flare-up phases and that clinical remissions can occur spontaneously or with treatment [1–5].

A great limit in the management of psoriasis, reported not only in adults but also in children and adolescents, is the low adherence to prescribed therapies, especially to topical treatments.

A practical tool that could be able to increase the patient's adherence to treatment and to monitor the efficacy and safety of prescribed therapies is to time and schedule a regular program of follow-up medical visit [6–10].

There are currently no standardized guidelines for therapies of childhood psoriasis; treatment approach is primarily based on guidelines, published expert opinions, and recommendations for adult psoriasis or experiences with systemic drugs acquired in other pediatric skin or inflammatory disorders.

The possibilities of psoriasis treatments have been expanded in the last years, with multiple available topical and systemic agents, although off-label therapies remain still widely used in pediatric psoriasis [8–11].

Evaluating the treatment of psoriasis in children, several factors should be considered, such as the age of the child, the impact on quality of life due to the disease, the involved body areas, the severity of psoriasis, and also the preferences of patient, in particular about application modalities of topical treatments (Table 7.1).

Table 7.1 Topical and systemic treatments of psoriasis in children

	Main characteristics
Topical treatments	
Keratolytic agents	• Urea, salicylic acid • Reduce and remove the superficial hyperkeratosis of psoriatic skin lesions • In infants the use of topical salicylic acid should be avoided as its topical application can lead to percutaneous salicylism
Topical corticosteroids	• Recommended topical corticosteroids in children: mometasone furoate 0.1%, methylprednisolone aceponate 0.1% • The use of high-potency corticosteroids in children should be limited for short periods of treatment (no more than 2 weeks) or in areas of thick skin (such as palms and soles) • Particular attention should be paid to the use of topical corticosteroids in sensitive areas, such as face and anogenital regions
Topical vitamin D analogues/vitamin D analogues combined with topical corticosteroids	• Topical vitamin D derivatives act inhibiting keratinocyte proliferation • Combination of vitamin D analogues with topical corticosteroids leads to drug synergy and to a steroid-sparing effect • There are available several compounded topical formulations containing calcipotriol and betamethasone dipropionate, with a good profile of efficacy and safety
Topical calcineurin inhibitors	• Approved for the treatment of atopic dermatitis in children, so their use for pediatric psoriasis is off-label tacrolimus (0.03%/0.1% ointment) and pimecrolimus (0.03% ointment) • Promote the clearance of psoriatic skin lesions, inhibiting cytokine production by T-lymphocytes, reducing skin inflammation and limiting T cells proliferation
Systemic treatments	
Oral retinoids	• Off-label for the treatment of pediatric psoriasis • Oral retinoids act with an antiproliferative mechanism, favoring the differentiation of epidermal keratinocytes and with anti-inflammatory effect • Recommended dosage: 0.3–0.5 mg/kg/day • Full blood count, liver enzymes, serum creatinine, pregnancy test (urine), fasting blood sugar, triglycerides/cholesterol/HDL are recommended every 4 weeks during treatment • An effective contraception 1 month before starting therapy, throughout the duration of treatment and up to 3 years after the end of treatment is recommended
Cyclosporine	• Off-label for the treatment of pediatric psoriasis • Immunosuppressive properties (immunosuppression) • Monitoring of blood pressure and several laboratory tests (creatinine, uric acid, liver enzymes, bilirubin, alkaline phosphatase, potassium, magnesium, urinalysis, complete blood count) are recommended every 4 weeks during treatment • Recommended dosage: 2.5–5 mg/kg/day

Table 7.1 (continued)

	Main characteristics
Methotrexate	• Off-label for the treatment of pediatric psoriasis • Methotrexate is an analogue of folic acid, it competitively inhibits the enzyme dihydrofolate reductase, the thymidylate and purine synthesis, resulting in decreased synthesis of DNA and RNA of activated T cells and keratinocytes; methotrexate has an antiproliferative and immunomodulatory effects • Laboratory tests (blood count, liver enzymes, creatinine, urine sediment, urine pregnancy test in females of child-bearing age, serology for HBV/HCV and serum albumin) are recommended • Recommended dosage: 0.2–0.7 mg/kg once a week
Biologic agents	
Etanercept	• A human dimeric fusion protein which binds to soluble TNF-α • Approved as treatment of severe, chronic plaque psoriasis in children (≥6 to 18 years old according to EMA; ≥4 to 18 years old according to FDA) after inadequate response or intolerance to conventional systemic treatments or phototherapy • Full blood count, liver enzymes, serum creatinine, urine analysis, pregnancy test (urine), HBV/HCV, HIV (prior to therapy), tuberculosis screening including chest X-ray (prior to therapy) are recommended • Subcutaneous administration • Recommended dosage: 0.8 mg/kg once a week
Adalimumab	• A recombinant human immunoglobulin G1 (IgG1) monoclonal antibody which binds to soluble TNF-α • Approved as first-line therapy for the treatment of severe chronic plaque psoriasis in children (≥4 to 18 years old) who are inappropriate candidates for topical treatments and phototherapies or have had an inadequate response • Serology for HBV/HCV, HIV and tuberculosis screening including chest X-ray are recommended before starting treatment; monitoring of blood count, liver enzymes, serum creatinine, urine sediment, and urine pregnancy test during treatment is recommended • Subcutaneous administration • Recommended dosage: An initial dose of 20 mg followed by a subsequent dose of 20 mg after 7 days, then a dosage of 20 mg every 2 weeks (children under 30 kg); an initial dose of 40 mg, followed by a subsequent dose of 40 mg after 7 days, then continuing with 40 mg every 2 weeks (children over 30 kg)

(continued)

Table 7.1 (continued)

	Main characteristics
Ustekinumab	• A human monoclonal antibody targeting the p40 subunit of interleukin-12/23 • Approved for the treatment of moderate-to-severe plaque psoriasis in children and adolescents above the age of 6 years of age whose condition has not improved or who have contraindications to systemic conventional treatments (such as methotrexate and cyclosporine) or to phototherapy • Subcutaneous administration • Recommended dosage: an initial dose of 0.75 mg/kg (children under 60 kg) or 45 mg (children over 60 kg), followed by an equal dose after 4 weeks, then every 12 weeks • Serology for HBV/HCV, HIV and tuberculosis screening including chest X-ray are recommended before starting treatment; monitoring of blood count, liver enzymes, serum creatinine, urine sediment, and urine pregnancy test during treatment is recommended
Secukinumab	• Human monoclonal antibody that directly inhibits interleukin-17A (IL-17A) • Approved for the treatment of moderate-to-severe plaque psoriasis in children and adolescents aged >6 years who are candidates for systemic treatments • Subcutaneous administration • Recommended dosage: 75 mg (for children up to 50 kg) and 150 mg (for children weighing more than 50 kg) with an initial dose at weeks 0, 1, 2, 3 and 4, followed by monthly maintenance dosing
Ixekizumab	• Ixekizumab is a fully human monoclonal antibody that inhibits the signal of IL-17 • Subcutaneous administration • FDA approved ixekizumab for the treatment of severe plaque psoriasis in children aged ≥6 years (not approved by the EMA for children with weight under 25 kg) • Recommended dosage: initial dose of 40 mg and 20 mg thereafter (children up to 25 kg), initial dose of 80 mg and 40 mg thereafter (children ≥25 to ≤50 kg), initial dose of 160 mg and 80 mg thereafter (children ≥50 kg) • Ixekizumab is administered every 4 weeks

7.1 Topical Treatments

For the treatment of mild-to-moderate localized psoriasis, topical therapies represent the first-line treatment in children.

Available vehicles include creams, foams, gels, ointments, and lotions.

Thicker vehicles (such as ointments) are generally more effective, although the location of involved areas and preference of patient should ultimately guide the prescription of treatment by physicians. Lotions and gels are generally preferred in case of scalp involvement while ointment or spray should be preferred for dry and wide surface involved areas.

Topical treatments include topical corticosteroids, vitamin D analogues, and topical products with a combination of these agents.

Some simple agents commonly used in pediatric psoriasis also include keratolytic agents (such as salicylic acid and urea), which act reducing and removing the typical superficial hyperkeratosis of psoriatic skin lesions. Particular attention should be paid to the use of salicylic acid, as its topical application can lead to percutaneous salicylism in infants, so in this age group the use of topical salicylic acid should be avoided [12, 13].

Other topical agents used in pediatric psoriasis are calcineurin inhibitors, such as tacrolimus and pimecrolimus, which seem to show a good profile of efficacy and safety [1, 5, 12–19].

However, most of topical agents usually prescribed for the treatment of pediatric psoriasis require an off-label prescribing, as they are not officially approved for pediatric use [11].

7.1.1 Topical Corticosteroids

In all age group of patients, the most commonly prescribed topical treatments of psoriasis are topical corticosteroids.

The most common used corticosteroids in children are low-to medium-potency corticosteroids, such as mometasone furoate 0.1% and methylprednisolone aceponate 0.1%.

The choice of topical corticosteroids in pediatric psoriasis should mainly consider the skin areas involved [1, 4, 5, 9, 12–14].

Low potency steroids are generally used for more sensitive areas, such as face, head, neck, and anogenital regions. Moderate potency steroids are commonly used on the scalp and extremities.

In children, the use of high-potency corticosteroids should be limited for short periods of treatment (no more than 2 weeks) or in areas of thick skin (such as palms and soles).

Potential adverse local events related to the prolonged use of topical corticosteroids in adults are skin atrophy/striae, telangiectasias, hypertrichosis, and acneiform eruptions, so particular attention should be paid to the use of topical corticosteroids in pediatric age, especially in sensitive areas, such as face and anogenital regions [1, 4, 5, 9, 12–14].

7.1.2 Topical Vitamin D Analogues/Vitamin D Analogues Combined with Topical Corticosteroids

Topical vitamin D analogues, such as calcipotriol and calcitriol, are commonly used in children with psoriasis, showing a good profile of efficacy and safety. The most common adverse events of topical vitamin D derivatives are local skin irritation and itching, so the use of these agents should be avoided on sensitive areas, such as face and anogenital regions.

Topical vitamin D analogues are not recommended in children under the age of 2 years.

Topical vitamin D derivatives are also often prescribed in combination with topical corticosteroids for the treatment of psoriasis in children. Topical vitamin D derivatives act inhibiting keratinocyte proliferation and their combination with topical corticosteroids leads to drug synergy and to a steroid-sparing effect [20–23].

Currently there are available several compounded topical formulations containing calcipotriol and betamethasone dipropionate, which generally show a good profile of efficacy and safety.

7.1.3 Topical Calcineurin Inhibitors

Topical calcineurin inhibitors (such as tacrolimus and pimecrolimus) are other topical agents used in the treatment of pediatric psoriasis. These agents are able to promote the clearance of psoriatic skin lesions, as they inhibit cytokine production by T-lymphocytes, reducing skin inflammation and limiting T cells proliferation.

Both tacrolimus (in formulation at 0.03%/0.1% ointment) and pimecrolimus (in formulation at 0.03% ointment) are approved for the treatment of atopic dermatitis in children, so their use for pediatric psoriasis is off-label. Although a black box warning due to a theoretical increased risk of skin cancer and lymphoma, topical calcineurin inhibitors generally show a good profile of efficacy and safety, avoiding the risk of skin atrophy and allowing their use in sensitive areas (such as anogenital regions and face) [24, 25].

7.2   Phototherapy

An alternative physical treatment for pediatric psoriasis is represented by phototherapy.

Phototherapy is available as narrowband ultraviolet B light (nb-UVB) or UVA in association with psoralen (PUVA). However, PUVA therapy was reported and associated with an increased risk of carcinogenesis in adult patients with psoriasis, so nb-UVB (311 cm) is the treatment of choice for the treatment of psoriasis both in adults and in children [26–29].

Nb-UVB-phototherapy acts inhibiting T-cell activation, epidermal hyperproliferation, and with an anti-angiogenic effect.

Nb-UVB-phototherapy should be considered in children with plaque-type and guttate psoriasis with extensive involved body areas or poorly controlled with topical treatments. Mean duration of phototherapy is generally 2–3 months with an average of two sessions per week [10–14, 26–29].

Some common limits of phototherapy for the child and parents are related to logistics and frequency of medical appointments, which often result difficult for many families with busy schedules.

Therefore, determining if a child is a good candidate for phototherapy, several factors should be evaluated, such as assessment of history, unsuccessful previous treatments, ability and possibility of the family to go to the hospital frequently [26–29].

Considering that there are no official guidelines on the age of child which phototherapy can be started and that clinical experiences are lacking for children under the age of 8 years, an age of 8–10 years could be a rational cut-off to consider phototherapy in pediatric patients with psoriasis, also considering that a young child could not be able to remain still for the length of therapeutic session in the lamp booth [10–14, 26–29].

Common short-term adverse effects of phototherapy include erythema, itching, burning, and blistering.

7.3 Systemic Treatments

Systemic treatments in children with psoriasis are usually reserved for those patients resistant to topical treatments, with extensive body surface area involvement and with significant impairment in quality of life.

All conventional systemic drugs for the treatment of psoriasis in adults (retinoids, cyclosporine, and methotrexate) are off-label in children.

7.3.1 Retinoids

Systemic retinoids are actually not approved for use in pediatric psoriasis because of a lack of clinical trials. Among retinoids, acitretin is approved for the treatment of psoriasis in adults, but very few data are available about acitretin in children. Case reports and case series report the use of acitretin in children with generalized or localized pustular psoriasis.

Systemic retinoids act with an antiproliferative mechanism, favoring the differentiation of epidermal keratinocytes and with anti-inflammatory effect.

Acitretin dosages varied, according to the patients' age and weight, from 0.3 to 0.5 mg/kg daily for 4 weeks, to 0.5–0.8 mg/kg daily for 2–6 months [5, 12–17].

The most common adverse effects of acitretin include cheilitis, xerosis, skin fragility, epistaxis, hair loss, and dry eyes and are generally transient and dose dependent. In patients under treatment with acitretin, laboratory follow-up is needed to monitor liver enzymes, the lipid profile, and renal function. Due to the high teratogenicity and to the slow clearance of oral retinoids, their use in female adolescents should be carefully considered [5, 12–17].

An effective contraception 1 month before starting therapy, throughout the duration of treatment and up to 3 years after the end of treatment and monthly controls of blood beta-human chorionic gonadotropin levels should be recommended in female adolescents under treatment with oral retinoids [5, 12–17, 30].

7.3.2 Cyclosporine

Cyclosporine is not currently approved in childhood psoriasis as very few data are available in literature. Cyclosporine has an immunosuppressant action, inhibiting cytokine signaling by lymphocyte involved in the pathogenesis of psoriasis.

Treatment with cyclosporine could be justified only for carefully selected and strictly monitored children with severe flairs of psoriasis when other treatments have failed.

Although there is no consensus on dosage and time of use of cyclosporine in the pediatric population, the initial dose of cyclosporine in children is usually between 2.5 and 5 mg/kg/day. Due to the few available data about dosing, efficacy, and safety of cyclosporine in children, the lowest possible dose and shortest treatment period are recommended.

Due to the most common adverse effects of cyclosporine which are related to a possible increase in blood pressure and to a potential renal toxicity, close monitoring of blood pressure and renal function is required [5, 12–17, 31, 32].

7.3.3 Methotrexate

Methotrexate is not currently approved in pediatric psoriasis as very few data are available. In children, methotrexate is only approved for the treatment of juvenile idiopathic arthritis, inflammatory bowel disease, and malignancies.

Methotrexate is an analogue of folic acid, it competitively inhibits the enzyme dihydrofolate reductase, the thymidylate and purine synthesis, resulting in decreased synthesis of DNA and RNA of activated T cells and keratinocytes; methotrexate also has antiproliferative and immunomodulatory effects.

About use of methotrexate for the treatment of psoriasis in children, only small case series and case reports are available in literature. According to the experts' opinion, methotrexate is considered to be the traditional systemic treatment of choice in severe, recalcitrant plaque-type and guttate psoriasis in children [5, 12–17, 33].

The most common adverse events in patients under treatment with methotrexate are mild to severe nausea and vomiting, but hepatotoxicity and hematologic toxicity are other potential side effects rarely observed. Therefore, routine monitoring of blood counts and liver function tests are recommended in children under treatment with methotrexate [5, 12–17, 33].

Although there is no consensus on dosage and time of use of methotrexate in the pediatric population, the dose usually given varies from 0.2 to 0.7 mg/kg once a week. As soon as therapeutic control is achieved, the dose should be gradually reduced to an effective but lower maintenance dose.

7.4   Biologic Treatments

Biologic agents are relatively new drugs which target specific mediators of the inflammatory cascade in psoriasis. Biologic agents generally offer more favorable dosing regimens and require less frequent laboratory test monitoring than conventional systemic therapies.

Biologic drugs are reserved to children with severe plaque-type psoriasis resistant to conventional treatments although conventional therapies are not approved for the treatment of pediatric psoriasis. All patients should be screened for tuberculosis and for HBV/HCV,HIV infection and laboratory studies before initiating therapy [5, 12–17, 34–37].

Most common adverse events of biologic agents are associated with infectious diseases (such as opportunistic infections, reactivation of latent tuberculosis) and malignancies, in particular lymphomas, although these events are very rare.

Among biologic agents, etanercept, adalimumab, ustekinumab, and secukinumab currently have approval by European Medicines Agency for the treatment of moderate-to-severe chronic plaque psoriasis in children.

7.4.1   Etanercept

Etanercept is a human dimeric fusion protein which binds to soluble TNF-α.

Etanercept is approved for the treatment of severe, chronic plaque psoriasis in children ($\geq$6 to 18 years old according to EMA; $\geq$4 to 18 years old according to FDA) after inadequate response or intolerance to conventional systemic treatments or phototherapy.

Etanercept should be considered as a second-line drug in severe plaque psoriasis in children although no conventional first-line treatments are approved in the pediatric population.

Etanercept is administered subcutaneously and the recommended dosage for the treatment of psoriasis in children is of 0.8 mg/kg once a week (to a maximum of 50 mg/week).

The most commonly reported adverse events of etanercept are upper respiratory tract infection, nasopharyngitis, headache, and injection-site reactions [5, 12–17, 38].

Before starting treatment with etanercept, serology for HBV/HCV, HIV, and tuberculosis screening including chest X-ray are recommended.

7.4.2   Adalimumab

Adalimumab is a recombinant human immunoglobulin G1 (IgG1) monoclonal antibody which binds to soluble TNF-α.

Adalimumab is approved as first-line therapy for the treatment of severe chronic plaque psoriasis in children (≥4 years old) who are inappropriate candidates for topical treatments and phototherapies or have had an inadequate response.

Adalimumab is administered subcutaneously and the recommended dosage for the treatment of severe plaque psoriasis in children varies based on the weight of child. In children weighing less than 30 kg, the dosing schedule includes an initial dose of 20 mg, followed by a subsequent dose of 20 mg after 7 days, than a dosage of 20 mg every 2 weeks.

In children with weight ≥30 kg, the adalimumab dosing schedule includes an initial dose of 40 mg, followed by a subsequent dose of 40 mg after 7 days, then continuing with 40 mg every 2 weeks [5, 12–17, 39].

The most common adverse events of adalimumab are infections of the upper respiratory tract (e.g., nasopharyngitis and pharyngitis) and injection-site reactions.

Before starting treatment with adalimumab, serology for HBV/HCV, HIV, and tuberculosis screening including chest X-ray are recommended. Monitoring of blood count, liver enzymes, serum creatinine, urine sediment, and urine pregnancy test during treatment is recommended.

7.4.3 Ustekinumab

Ustekinumab is a fully human monoclonal antibody targeting the p40 subunit of interleukin-12/23.

Ustekinumab is approved for the treatment of moderate-to-severe plaque psoriasis in children and adolescents (≥6 years old) whose condition has not improved or who have contraindications to systemic conventional treatments (such as methotrexate and cyclosporine) or to phototherapy [5, 12–17].

Ustekinumab is administered subcutaneously and the recommended dosage for the treatment of severe plaque psoriasis in children varies based on the weight of child.

The dosing schedule includes an initial dose of 0.75 mg/kg (in children weighing less than 60 kg) or 45 mg (in children weighing more than 60 kg), followed by an equal dose after 4 weeks, then every 12 weeks [5, 12–17].

The most common adverse events of ustekinumab are infections of the upper respiratory tract (e.g., nasopharyngitis and pharyngitis), headache and injection-site reactions.

Before starting treatment with ustekinumab, serology for HBV/HCV, HIV, and tuberculosis screening including chest X-ray are recommended.

7.4.4 Secukinumab

Secukinumab is a fully human monoclonal antibody that directly inhibits interleukin-17A (IL-17A), a cytokine involved in the pathogenesis of moderate-to-severe plaque psoriasis.

Secukinumab is approved in 2020 by EMA for the treatment of moderate-to-severe plaque psoriasis in children and adolescents aged ≥6 years who are candidates for systemic treatments. FDA did not approve secukinumab for the treatment of psoriasis in children.

Secukinumab is administered subcutaneously with an initial dose at weeks 0, 1, 2, 3, and 4, followed by monthly maintenance dosing. The recommended dose is 75 mg (for children up to 50 kg) and 150 mg (for children weighing more than 50 kg) [5, 12–17].

7.4.5 Ixekizumab

Ixekizumab is a fully human monoclonal antibody that inhibits the signal of IL-17.

Ixekizumab is not approved by the EMA for children with weight under 25 kg.

FDA approved ixekizumab for the treatment of severe plaque psoriasis in children aged ≥6 years at different dosage according to the weight of the child: for children weighing less than 25 kg, ixekizumab is approved at an initial dose of 40 mg and 20 mg thereafter. In children with weight ≥25 to ≤50 kg, ixekizumab is approved at an initial dose of 80 mg and 40 mg thereafter. In children with weight ≥50 kg, ixekizumab is approved at an initial dose of 160 mg and 80 mg thereafter. Ixekizumab is administered subcutaneously every 4 weeks [5, 12–17].

7.4.6 Other Biologic Treatments and Small-Molecules Drugs

Guselkumab, tildrakizumab, and risankizumab are monoclonal antibodies which inhibit IL-23, all approved for the treatment of moderate-to-severe psoriasis in adult patients.

The lack of data for the treatment of psoriasis in children is now being addressed, as these biologic drugs are being evaluated in phase II/III clinical trials that are recruiting patients aged ≥6 to <18 years [5, 14–16].

Brodalumab (a human monoclonal antibodies which inhibits the signal of IL-17) is another biologic drug which is currently being evaluated with several phase II/III clinical trials or the treatment of plaque psoriasis in the pediatric population.

About small-molecules drugs, apremilast is an oral PDE4 inhibitor already approved for the treatment of moderate-to-severe plaque psoriasis and psoriatic arthritis in adult patients; apremilast is now being evaluated in phase II/III clinical trials that are recruiting patients aged ≥ 6 to <18 years with moderate-to-severe plaque psoriasis [5, 14–16, 40].

7.5   Therapeutic Education and Pro-active Treatment

The therapeutic objectives for a child with psoriasis should be multidimensional, including management of clinical flare-ups, prevention of exacerbation, maintenance of remission and prevention of long-term complications, also considering the possible comorbidities and the impact on quality of life [41–43].

In this context, therapeutic education plays a key role. Physicians should give exhaustive explanations about the treatment of psoriasis, but they should also make sure that children and parents really understand the pathophysiology, course, types of available treatments, etc. of psoriasis and its management, optimizing compliance with the therapeutic objectives.

Physicians should clearly explain to parents and adolescents that the pathogenesis of psoriasis is based on genetic and immunological factors, that the disease is chronic with an alternation of remissions and flare-up phases and that remissions can occur spontaneously or with treatment [41].

Child and parents should also know that several environmental factors (including mental, physical stress, infections, mechanical trauma, etc.) could act as trigger factors, inducing the clinical exacerbation phases of psoriasis.

Mental stress is a common trigger factor in pediatric age although often underestimated. Stress is very common in children, generally related to the anxiety due to school or sports activities and performances or related to familial conditions (such as parental separation, the birth of a younger brother, and many other factors) [41–43].

Studies suggest that the stress factor plays a greater role in children than in adults in the onset of exacerbations of psoriasis. In some cases, psychological support could be necessary and should be recommended.

The short-term benefits of treatments and long-term remission between flare-up phases can be often difficult to achieve, requiring a long-term treatment strategies in the management of pediatric psoriasis [41].

A "pro-active" therapeutic approach could be beneficial, trying to anticipate disease progression, to limit its severity and the occurrence of new exacerbation phases.

The first "pro-active" therapeutic approach is the classic "gradual withdrawal" of topical treatment over a period of several months in order to avoid or delay flare-up phases.

Another "pro-active" therapeutic approach is "weekend therapy": topical treatments are applied to the usually affected areas on Saturday and Sunday only (or on two separate weekdays), in order to reduce the frequency of clinical flare-ups [41, 42].

The application of topical emollients is also essential, reducing the frequency of relapse and increasing the duration of remission phases. In addition, a regular use of emollients is able to reduce itching, limiting the risk of scratching and of Koebner phenomenon on dry skin [41, 42].

References

1. Bronckers IM, Paller AS, van Geel MJ, van de Kerkhof PC, Seyger MM. Psoriasis in children and adolescents: diagnosis. Management and comorbidities. Paediatr Drugs. 2015;17(5):373–84.
2. Shah KN. Diagnosis and treatment of pediatric psoriasis: current and future. Am J Clin Dermatol. 2013;14(3):195–213.
3. Stahle M, Atakan N, Boehncke WH, et al. Juvenile psoriasis and its clinical management: a European expert group consensus. J Ger Soc Dermatol. 2010;8(10):812–8.
4. Fotiadou C, Lazaridou E, Ioannides D. Management of psoriasis in adolescence. Adolesc Health Med Ther. 2014;5:25–34.
5. Tolliver S, Pepper AN, Pothiawala S, Silverberg NB. Pediatric psoriasis. In: Weinberg JM, Lebwohl M, editors. Advances in psoriasis. Cham: Springer; 2021.
6. Luersen K, Davis SA, Kaplan SG, Abel TD, Winchester WW, Feldman SR. Sticker charts: a method for improving adherence to treatment of chronic diseases in children. Pediatr Dermatol. 2012;29(4):403–8.
7. Boehncke WH, Schön MP. Psoriasis Lancet. 2015;386(9997):983–94. https://doi.org/10.1016/S0140-6736(14)61909-711.
8. Mahé E. Childhood psoriasis. Eur J Dermatol. 2016;26(6):537–48.
9. Tollefson MM. Diagnosis and management of psoriasis in children. Pediatr Clin N Am. 2014;61(2):261–77.
10. Davis SA, Lin HC, Yu CH, Balkrishnan R, Feldman SR. Underuse of early follow-up visits: a missed opportunity to improve patients' adherence. J Drugs Dermatol JDD. 2014;13(7):833–6.
11. Haulrig MB, Zachariae C, Skov L. Off-label treatments for pediatric psoriasis: lessons for the clinic. Psoriasis (Auckl). 2021;11:1–20.
12. Mahé E. Optimal management of plaque psoriasis in adolescents: current perspectives. Psoriasis (Auckl). 2020;27(10):45–56.
13. Kravvas G, Gholam K. Use of topical therapies for pediatric psoriasis: a systematic review. Pediatr Dermatol. 2018;35(3):296–302.
14. Menter A, Cordoro KM, Davis DMR, et al. Joint American Academy of Dermatology–National psoriasis foundation guidelines of care for the management and treatment of psoriasis in pediatric patients. J Am Acad Dermatol 2020;82(1):161–201.
15. Nogueira M, Paller AS, Torres T. Targeted therapy for Pediatric psoriasis. Paediatr Drugs. 2021;23(3):203–12.
16. Fortina AB, Bardazzi F, Berti S, et al. Treatment of severe psoriasis in children: recommendations of an Italian expert group. Eur J Pediatr. 2017;176(10):1339–54.
17. De Jager ME, de Jong EM, van de Kerkhof PC, Seyger MM. Efficacy and safety of treatments for childhood psoriasis: a systematic literature review. J Am Acad Dermatol. 2010;62:1013–30.
18. Bhutani T, Kamangar F, Cordoro KM. Management of pediatric psoriasis. Pediatr Ann. 2012;41(1):e1–7.
19. Silverberg NB. Update on pediatric psoriasis, part 2: therapeutic management. Cutis. 2010;86(4):172–6.
20. Lara-Corrales I, Xi N, Pope E. Childhood psoriasis treatment: evidence published over the last 5 years. Rev Recent Clin Trials. 2011;6(1):36–43.
21. van Geel MJ, Mul K, Oostveen AM, van de Kerkhof PC, de Jong EM, Seyger MM. Calcipotriol/betamethasone dipropionate ointment in mild-to-moderate paediatric psoriasis: long-term daily clinical practice data in a prospective cohort. Br J Dermatol. 2014;171(2):363–9.
22. Gooderham M, Debarre JM, Keddy-Grant J, Xu Z, Kurvits M, Goodfield M. Safety and efficacy of calcipotriol plus betamethasone dipropionate gel in the treatment of scalp psoriasis in adolescents 12–17 years of age. Br J Dermatol. 2014;171(6):1470–7.
23. Oostveen AM, de Jong EM, Donders AR, van de Kerkhof PC, Seyger MM. Treatment of paediatric scalp psoriasis with calcipotriene/betamethasone dipropionate scalp formulation: effectiveness, safety and influence on children's quality of life in daily practice. J Eur Acad Dermatol Venereol JEADV. 2015;29(6):1193–7.

24. Brune A, Miller DW, Lin P, Cotrim-Russi D, et al. Tacrolimus ointment is effective for psoriasis on the face and intertriginous areas in pediatric patients. Pediatr Dermatol. 2007;24(1):76–80.
25. U.S. Food and Drug Administration. Information for healthcare professionals: tacrolimus (marketed as protopic). 2005. Last updated 21 Jan 2010. http://www.fda.gov/Drugs/DrugSafety/PostmarketDrugSafetyInformationforPatientsandProviders/ucm126497.htm. Accessed 12 Oct 2011.
26. Zamberk P, Velazquez D, Campos M, Hernanz JM, Lazaro P. Paediatric psoriasis—narrowband UVB treatment. J Eur Acad Dermatol Venereol JEADV. 2010;24(4):415–9.
27. Pavlovsky M, Baum S, Shpiro D, Pavlovsky L, Pavlotsky F. Narrow band UVB: is it effective and safe for paediatric psoriasis and atopic dermatitis? J Eur Acad Dermatol Venereol JEADV. 2011;25(6):727–9.
28. Jury CS, McHenry P, Burden AD, Lever R, Bilsland D. Narrowband ultraviolet B (UVB) phototherapy in children. Clin Exp Dermatol. 2006;31(2):196–9.
29. Veith W, Deleo V, Silverberg N. Medical phototherapy in childhood skin diseases. Minerva Pediatr. 2011;63(4):327–33.
30. Di Lernia V, Bonamonte D, Lasagni C, et al. Effectiveness and safety of acitretin in children with plaque psoriasis: a multicenter retrospective analysis. Pediatr Dermatol. 2016;33(5):530–5.
31. Di Lernia V, Stingeni L, Boccaletti V, et al. Effectiveness and safety of cyclosporine in pediatric plaque psoriasis: a multicentric retrospective analysis. J Dermatolog Treat. 2016;27(5):395–8.
32. Altomare G, Ayala F, Bardazzi F, et al. Cyclosporine in psoriasis: comparison of a 25-year real world Italian experience to current European guidelines. G Ital Dermatol Venereol. 2016;151:432–5.
33. Hashkes PJ, Becker ML, Cabral DA, et al. Methotrexate: new uses for an old drug. J Pediatr. 2014;164:231–6.
34. van Geel MJ, Mul K, de Jager ME, van de Kerkhof PC, de Jong EM, Seyger MM. Systemic treatments in paediatric psoriasis: a systematic evidence-based update. J Eur Acad Dermatol Venereol. 2015;29:425–37.
35. Marqueling AL, Cordoro KM. Systemic treatments for severe pediatric psoriasis: a practical approach. Dermatol Clin. 2013;31:267–88.
36. Charbit L, Mahé E, Phan A, et al. Groupe de Recherche de la Société Française de Dermatologie Pédiatrique. Systemic treatments in childhood psoriasis: a French multicentre study on 154 children. Br J Dermatol. 2016;174:1118–21.
37. Sticherling M, Augustin M, Boehncke WH, et al. Therapy of psoriasis in childhood and adolescence—a German expert consensus. J Ger Soc Dermatol. 2011;9(10):815–23.
38. Di Lernia V, Guarneri C, Stingeni L, et al. Effectiveness of etanercept in children with plaque psoriasis in real practice: a one-year multicenter retrospective study. J Dermatolog Treat. 2018;29(3):217–9.
39. Di Lernia V. Adalimumab for treating childhood plaque psoriasis: a clinical trial evaluation. Expert Opin Biol Ther. 2017;17(12):1553–6.
40. Smith R. Pediatric psoriasis treated with apremilast. JAAD Case Rep. 2016;2(1):89–91.
41. Lavaud J, Mahé E. Proactive treatment in childhood psoriasis. Ann Dermatol Venereol. 2020;147(1):29–35.
42. Man MQ, Ye L, Hu L, Jeong S, Elias PM, Lv C. Improvements in epidermal function prevent relapse of psoriasis: a self-controlled study. Clin Exp Dermatol. 2019;44(6):654–7.
43. Randa H, Todberg T, Skov L, Larsen LS, Zachariae R. Health-related quality of life in children and adolescents with psoriasis: a systematic review and meta-analysis. Acta Derm Venereol. 2017;97(5):555–63.

Comorbidities

8

Psoriasis is associated with several systemic diseases in adults, and more and more real-world evidence are available about the association of the same comorbidities with psoriasis also in children. Cardiovascular and metabolic diseases are the principal systemic comorbidities of psoriasis both in adults and children. The concept of the "psoriatic march" could explain the association between these comorbidities and psoriasis, as the systemic and chronic inflammation in psoriasis may cause insulin resistance, triggering endothelial cell dysfunction and leading to atherosclerosis and increasing the risk of myocardial infarction and stroke (Fig. 8.1) [1–7].

On the other hand, in over-weight and obese patients with psoriasis the systemic inflammation is further increased as the adipose tissue acts as an endocrine tissue, releasing pro-inflammatory cytokines.

Over-weight/obesity, central obesity, hypertension, hyperlipidemia, diabetes mellitus, and metabolic syndrome have been found associated with psoriasis in children and adolescents.

Therefore, a special attention should be given by pediatricians and dermatologists to the screening and monitoring the parameters related to these metabolic and cardiovascular comorbidities in children with psoriasis, in order to early identify and manage them (Table 8.1).

Furthermore, children with psoriasis also have a high risk of developing other diseases, such as arthritis, psychiatric comorbidities, and gastrointestinal diseases, which are associated with psoriasis.

© The Author(s), under exclusive license to Springer Nature
Switzerland AG 2022
A. Belloni Fortina, F. Caroppo, *Pediatric Psoriasis*,
https://doi.org/10.1007/978-3-030-90712-9_8

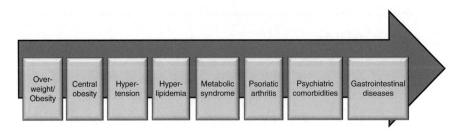

Fig 8.1 A summary scheme of systemic comorbidities of psoriasis, involved in the so-called psoriatic march

Table 8.1 Comorbidities associated with childhood psoriasis and relative screening recommendations

Comorbidities	Screening recommendation
Over-weight, obesity, and central obesity	• Yearly screening using BMI and WHtR (children >2 years old); • Recommendations: Lifestyle changes (diet and physical activity); • Refer to a pediatric endocrinologist or dietician.
Diabetes and metabolic syndrome	• Yearly screening using fasting serum glucose; • Recommendations: Lifestyle changes (diet and physical activity); • Refer to a pediatric endocrinologist.
Hypertension	• Yearly high BP screening using age, sex, and height reference charts (children >3 years old); • Recommendations: Lifestyle changes (diet and physical activity).
Hyperlipidemia	• Yearly screening using a fasting lipid panel.
Arthritis	• Complete physical examination; • Complete review of symptoms related to arthritis; • Refer to a pediatric rheumatologist.
Psychiatric comorbidities	• Yearly screening for depression, anxiety, and substance use.
Gastrointestinal diseases	• Complete medical and familial history collection; • Complete physical examination; • Complete review of gastrointestinal symptoms; • Refer to a pediatric gastroenterologist.

BMI Body Mass Index, *WHtR* waist to height ratio, *BP* blood pressure

8.1   Over-Weight, Obesity and Central Obesity

Children with psoriasis are at higher risk of being over-weight or obese.

Multiple studies have demonstrated increased odds of psoriasis in over-weight or obese children although the direction of causation is still not fully understood.

The calculation of Body Mass Index (BMI—weight in kilograms divided by height in meters squared) is a simple tool useful to determine the status of normal-, over-weight, or obesity of the child.

A child is over-weight when BMI is ≥85th percentile to <95th percentile for age and sex, and obese when BMI is ≥95th percentile [8].

In children with psoriasis, a yearly screening for over-weight and obesity using BMI percentile is recommended, starting at 2 years of age [9–13].

Central obesity (also known as "abdominal obesity") refers to the abdominal fat mass and it is a condition related to an excessive of visceral fat around the stomach.

Central obesity is a relevant parameter, as it has been strongly related to cardio-vascular and metabolic diseases, including an altered lipid profile, high blood pressure, and impaired glucose tolerance and insulin sensitivity, which have been reported to originate early in childhood.

Several studies found a correlation between psoriasis and central obesity in children. A common tool that could be used in children with psoriasis in order to assess and to determine central obesity is the Waist to Height Ratio (WHtR). WHtR is the value resulted dividing waist circumference by height, both measured in the same units. Central obesity is defined when WHtR is ≥0.5 [1–5, 14–16].

Central obesity seems to be associated with psoriasis in over-weight and obese children, comparing children with psoriasis with psoriasis-free children. Furthermore, central obesity seems to be associated with psoriasis also in normal-weight children, suggesting that this condition is correlated to psoriasis independently from the weight of patient [14].

WHtR and central obesity are considered parameters strictly related to the metabolic condition and to the risk of developing metabolic diseases, suggesting that they could represent a strong link between psoriasis and the risk of metabolic and cardiovascular comorbidities.

There is also an association between weight and severity of psoriasis, as weight seems increasing with psoriasis severity, with some evidence showing that adiposity could precede psoriatic lesions by 2 years in a majority of children with psoriasis [4, 5].

In children with over-weight, obesity, or central obesity, physicians should discuss with patients and families the importance of performing lifestyle changes in order to minimize any additional cardiovascular and metabolic risk, also considering that psoriasis alone has been found to be an independent risk factor for cardiovascular diseases in adulthood.

Furthermore, lifestyle changes may reduce not only BMI, improving the status of over-weight or obesity, but also may improve the severity of psoriasis and the quality of life.

Obese children with psoriasis should be referred to an appropriate multidisciplinary child weight management center or dietician [9–13].

8.2 Hypertension

Several studies reported an association of hypertension and psoriasis in children [1–5, 16, 17].

Blood pressure values are categorized as normal blood pressure (>50 and ≤90th sex, age, and height specific percentile), elevated blood pressure (>90th sex, age, and height specific percentile), stage 1 hypertension (≥95th sex, age, and height specific percentile), and stage 2 hypertension (≥95th sex, age, and height specific percentile +12 mmHg) [18].

Hypertension in children with psoriasis seems to be independent of child's weight, as blood pressure values seem higher, not only in over-weight and obese children, but also in normal-weight children with psoriasis.

Therefore, routine counseling and surveillance of blood pressure by pediatricians and dermatologists in children with psoriasis are important, as an early diagnosis of hypertension could improve the management of patients in the primary care setting [9–13].

In fact, in children with an early diagnosis of hypertension, physicians should discuss with patients and families the importance of performing lifestyle changes, in order to avoid starting therapies with drugs and in order to minimize any additional cardiovascular and metabolic risk. The National Heart Lung and Blood Institute and the American Academy of Pediatrics recommend several management strategies, including diet and/or pharmacological interventions, according to the stage of hypertension [9–13].

Physicians should also consider that some systemic treatments of psoriasis (such as cyclosporine) may increase the risk of hypertension and are contraindicated in patients with hypertension.

Screen for hypertension in children with psoriasis should be performed yearly starting at 3 years of age, using age, sex, and height reference charts.

8.3   Hyperlipidemia

An association between hyperlipidemia and psoriasis has been reported in children and adolescents with psoriasis [1–5, 19].

Hyperlipidemia represents a relevant metabolic alteration that could arise early in childhood; a yearly lipid screening during the following 2 age ranges (9–11 years old and 17–21 years old) is recommended in children and adolescents with psoriasis.

Screening should be performed with a fasting lipid panel, which consists of total cholesterol level, low-density lipoprotein, cholesterol level, high-density lipoprotein cholesterol level, and triglycerides.

Pediatricians and dermatologists should also consider that some systemic treatments of psoriasis (such as oral retinoids) may increase the risk of hyperlipidemia and are contraindicated in patients with hyperlipidemia [9–13].

All children and their families should be educated about the association between psoriasis and dyslipidemia.

8.4   Diabetes and Metabolic Syndrome

An increased risk for insulin resistance, type 2 diabetes mellitus, and metabolic syndrome is correlated with psoriasis in adults [3, 20].

Recent studies found similar results in pediatric age; children with psoriasis seem at higher risk to develop diabetes mellitus and metabolic syndrome compared to healthy children [1, 2, 4–6, 21–23].

There are several recognized risk factors for type 2 diabetes that should be investigated in order to identify children with psoriasis at higher risk for insulin resistance and type 2 diabetes: maternal history of diabetes or gestational diabetes during the child's gestation, first- or second-degree relative with type 2 diabetes and race/ethnicity (Native American, African American, Latino, Asian American Pacific Islander).

Furthermore, a complete physical examination and a complete personal and family medical history in children with psoriasis should be always performed by pediatrician or dermatologist, in order to identify signs associated with insulin resistance or associated conditions, such as familial history of diabetes, acanthosis nigricans, hypertension, dyslipidemia, polycystic ovarian syndrome, small for gestational age birth weight.

Current screening guidelines for insulin resistance and type 2 diabetes mellitus are the same in children with and without psoriasis. It is recommended to screen every 3 years starting at age 10 years or at the onset of puberty in over-weight and obese children with psoriasis. The screening should be performed measuring fasting serum glucose [9–13].

For children with psoriasis and finding of high fasting serum glucose levels, lifestyle modifications, monitoring of blood glucose, and glycated hemoglobin are recommended and pharmacological therapy could be evaluated, referring the child to an endocrinologist.

Metabolic syndrome is a cluster of several medical conditions which occur together, and it is related to an increased risk of cardiovascular and metabolic diseases, such as heart disease, type 2 diabetes, and stroke [9–13].

Metabolic syndrome is diagnosed when at least three of the following five medical conditions are present: abdominal (or central) obesity, high blood pressure, high fasting blood glucose levels, high serum triglycerides levels, and low serum high-density lipoprotein (HDL) levels.

In pediatric age, metabolic syndrome has been defined by several studies which analyze levels for each component of metabolic syndrome, according to sex- and age- specific percentiles.

Two levels of metabolic syndrome are recognized in children: "monitoring level" (suggesting close monitoring of the child) and "action level" (suggesting the introduction of appropriate pediatric intervention), when the values of at least three of the five components are altered.

Waist circumference, blood pressure, triglycerides, and fasting blood glucose are considered altered in pediatric age with levels ≥90th sex- and age-specific percentile; HDL was considered altered with levels ≤10th sex- and age-specific percentile [24].

The increasing data about the association of metabolic syndrome and childhood psoriasis suggest that it is clinically very relevant to assess as soon as possible metabolic syndrome risk factors in children with psoriasis as they would probably benefit from lifestyle modifications in an effort to prevent cardiovascular diseases in adulthood [9–13].

8.5   Psoriatic Arthritis

Psoriatic arthritis is a form of arthritis or joint inflammation that affects both skin and joints.

Psoriatic arthritis causes joint pain and painful swelling, often affecting finger and toe joints; however, it can also affect wrists, ankles, knees, and the lower back.

This condition is most common in adults aged 30–50 years old, but it can start in childhood. In many cases, the skin disease starts before the arthritis. In children, psoriatic arthritis is a form of juvenile idiopathic arthritis.

Psoriatic arthritis occurs in a relatively small percentage of children (0.7–10.5%) and is less prevalent than in adults.

Psoriatic arthritis could be very destructive and debilitating and its early identification, diagnosis, and intervention in childhood are a priority, helping to ease pain and prevent joint damage from getting worse [10–13].

All children with psoriasis and their families should be educated about the risk of arthritis and should be educated to recognize its signs and symptoms.

Pediatricians and dermatologists should perform an adequate screening physical examination and a complete review of symptoms at each visit in children with psoriasis. In case of signs or symptoms related to psoriatic arthritis, the patient should be referred to a pediatric rheumatologist.

Clinical characteristics of psoriatic arthritis during the first peak (2–3 years of age) are similar to those of juvenile idiopathic arthritis, showing a female predisposition, antinuclear antibody positivity, and oligoarthritis or polyarthritis with a common small joint involvement. During the second peak (10–12 years of age), the characteristics seem to be more similar to spondyloarthritis: male predisposition, enthesitis, axial disease, and HLA-B27 positivity.

In pediatric psoriatic arthritis, the dactylitis (inflammation of an entire digit) is a common finding. Most of children with psoriatic arthritis develop arthritis 2 to 3 years prior to the onset of skin lesions, whereas adult patients tend to develop skin manifestations of psoriasis before arthritis symptoms.

Although several arthritis screening tools have been created for adult patients with psoriasis, none is actually validated in children.

However, some simple screening questions should be ask to the child and his parents in order to evaluate limp and stiffness, and to investigate joint pain (involving knees, ankles, wrists) particularly in the morning.

The most common symptoms of psoriatic arthritis that should be investigated in children with psoriasis are involvement of one or more joints, joint pain, tenderness or swelling, joint stiffness, which generally worse with rest and improve with movement [9–13].

Furthermore, physicians should be considered that there is a strong association between nail psoriasis involvement and the risk of psoriatic arthritis.

Nail involvement is found in up to 70% of patients with psoriatic arthritis. In particular, nail involvement may precede arthritis or may be considered as a predictor of future psoriatic joint damage. A possible explanation for this association could be the close anatomical link between the nail unit and the distal interphalangeal joint. Inflammation of the extensor tendon enthesis, that are the attachment points of ligaments, tendons, and joint capsules to bone, can extend to the nail unit and result in psoriatic nail alterations [9–13, 25].

Children with nail involvement should be always investigated for the presence of psoriatic arthritis.

Finally, physicians should consider that children with psoriasis and psoriatic arthritis have an increased risk for uveitis and should be screened routinely for it.

8.6 Psychiatric Comorbidities

While adults with psoriasis have a recognized increased risk of depression and other psychiatric disorders, limited studies investigated the incidence of psychiatric comorbidities among pediatric patients with psoriasis although increasing data are available about this topic in recent years [4].

Some studies were conducted in Europe and in USA, finding that children with psoriasis have higher risk for psychiatric diseases (such as depression, anxiety, and bipolar disease) compared with children without. Furthermore, these studies suggested that children with psoriasis may be at high risk for psychiatric treatment of psychiatric disorders. In fact, children with psoriasis are more often managed with psychotropic medications, including tricyclic antidepressant and anxiolytic drugs [4, 26].

The association between psoriasis and psychiatric diseases could be related to several factors; in fact, psoriasis often causes a social stigmatization since pediatric age, resulting in behavioral changes. On the other hand, depression could lead to increased risk behavior.

Considering the multidimensional impact of psoriasis on the life of children and adolescents, it should be also considered that psoriasis often confers a significant psychosocial disease burden, with an increased risk of several psychiatric disorders and subsequent treatment for psychiatric diseases, also in children [1, 2, 4–7, 26].

Considering the general widespread accessibility and low cost of psychiatric screening tools and the potentially serious consequences of untreated psychiatric diseases since from childhood, pediatricians and dermatologists should yearly screen children with psoriasis for depression, anxiety, and substance use, in order to early recognize psychiatric disorders and in order to allow an early treatment [9–13].

8.7 Gastrointestinal Diseases

Adult patients with psoriasis seem to be at higher risk to develop inflammatory bowel diseases (both Crohn disease and ulcerative colitis) and celiac disease.

A routinely screening including a complete medical and familial history collection and a complete physical examination should be performed in children with psoriasis, investigating weight loss, poor growth, and gastrointestinal symptoms (such as diarrhea and abdominal pain) [9–13].

In children with psoriasis and a decreased growth rate, an unexplained weight loss or symptoms consistent with inflammatory bowel disease or celiac disease (abdominal pain, nausea, vomiting, diarrhea), a formal gastrointestinal evaluation is recommended [9–13].

References

1. Phan K, Lee G, Fischer G. Pediatric psoriasis and association with cardiovascular and metabolic comorbidities: systematic review and meta-analysis. Pediatr Dermatol. 2020;37(4):661–9.
2. Bronckers IM, Paller AS, van Geel MJ, van de Kerkhof PC, Seyger MM. Psoriasis in children and adolescents: diagnosis. Management and comorbidities. Paediatr Drugs. 2015;17(5):373–84.
3. Jensen P, Skov L. Psoriasis and obesity. Dermatology. 2016;232:633–9.
4. Tolliver S, Pepper AN, Pothiawala S, Silverberg NB. Pediatric psoriasis. In: Weinberg JM, Lebwohl M, editors. Advances in psoriasis. Cham: Springer; 2021.
5. Tollefson MM, Van Houten HK, Asante D, Yao X, Maradit KH. Association of psoriasis with comorbidity development in children with psoriasis. JAMA Dermatol. 2018;154(3):286–92.
6. Edson-Heredia E, Anderson S, Guo J, et al. Real-world claims analyses of comorbidity burden. Treatment pattern: healthcare resource utilization, and costs in pediatric psoriasis. Adv Ther; 2021.
7. Tollefson MM. Diagnosis and management of psoriasis in children. Pediatr Clin N Am. 2014;61(2):261–77.
8. Centers for Disease Control and Prevention. (2018). Defining childhood obesity. Retrieved from https://www.cdc.gov/obesity/childhood/defining.html
9. Kang BY, O'Haver J, Andrews ID. Pediatric psoriasis comorbidities: screening recommendations for the primary care provider. J Pediatr Health Care. 2021;35(3):337–50.
10. Osier E, Wang AS, Tollefson MM, et al. Pediatric psoriasis comorbidity screening guidelines. JAMA Dermatol. 2017;153(7):698–704.
11. Ko SH, Chi CC, Yeh ML, Wang SH, Tsai YS, Hsu MY. Lifestyle changes for treating psoriasis. Cochrane Database Syst Rev. 2019;7(7):CD011972.
12. Elmets CA, Leonardi CL, Davis DMR, et al. Joint AAD-NPF guidelines of care for the management and treatment of psoriasis with awareness and attention to comorbidities. J Am Acad Dermatol. 2019;80(4):1073–113.
13. Menter A, Cordoro KM, Davis DMR, et al. Joint American Academy of Dermatology-National Psoriasis Foundation guidelines of care for the management and treatment of psoriasis in pediatric patients. J Am Acad Dermatol. 2020;82:161–201.
14. Guidolin L, Borin M, Fontana E, Caroppo F, Piaserico S, Fortina AB. Central obesity in children with psoriasis. Acta Derm Venereol. 2018;98(2):282–3.
15. Paller AS, Mercy K, Kwasny MJ, et al. Association of pediatric psoriasis severity with excess and central adiposity: an international cross-sectional study. JAMA Dermatol. 2013;149(2):166–76.
16. Paller A, Schenfeld J, Accortt NA, Kricorian G. A retrospective cohort study to evaluate the development of comorbidities, including psychiatric comorbidities, among a pediatric psoriasis population. Pediatr Dermatol. 2019;36:290–7.
17. Caroppo F, Ventura L, Belloni FA. High blood pressure in Normal-weight children with psoriasis. Acta Derm Venereol. 2019;99(3):329–30.

18. Flynn JT, Kaelber DC, Baker-Smith CM, Blowey D, Carroll AE, Daniels SR, et al. Clinical practice guideline for screening and management of high blood pressure in children and adolescents. Pediatrics. 2017;140:e20171904.
19. Koebnick C, Black MH, Smith N, et al. The association of psoriasis and elevated blood lipids in overweight and obese children. J Pediatr. 2011;159:577–83.
20. Azfar RS, Seminara NM, Shin DB, Troxel AB, Margolis DJ, Gelfand JM. Increased risk of diabetes mellitus and likelihood of receiving diabetes mellitus treatment in patients with psoriasis. Arch Dermatol. 2012;148:995–1000.
21. Au SC, Goldminz AM, Loo DS, et al. Association between pediatric psoriasis and the metabolic syndrome. J Am Acad Dermatol. 2021;66(6):1012–3.
22. Goldminz AM, Buzney CD, Kim N, et al. Prevalence of the metabolic syndrome in children with psoriatic disease. Pediatr Dermatol. 2013;30:700–5.
23. Caroppo F, Galderisi A, Ventura L, Belloni FA. Metabolic syndrome and insulin resistance in pre-pubertal children with psoriasis. Eur J Pediatr. 2021;180(6):1739–45.
24. Ahrens W, Moreno LA, Marild S, IDEFICS consortium, et al. Metabolic syndrome in young children: definition and results of the IDEFICS study. Int J Obes. 2014;38(Suppl 2):S4–S14.
25. Sobolewski P, Walecka I, Dopytalska K. Nail involvement in psoriatic arthritis. Reumatologia. 2017;55(3):131–5.
26. Kimball AB, Wu EQ, Guerin A, et al. Risks of developing psychiatric disorders in pediatric patients with psoriasis. J Am Acad Dermatol. 2012;67:651–657.e72.

Quality of Life

9

Psoriasis has a great impact on the quality of life and psychological well-being of children and adolescents.

In fact, representing the interface between the body and the external environment, the skin plays a key role in the delicate phase of building one's self-esteem, identity formation, and awareness of the subject [1–5].

Children are a vulnerable group of patients and psoriasis in pediatric age could greatly interfere with social relationships and with school and fun activities of children.

Several studies showed that skin disorders have a higher impact on quality of life compared to other diseases [5–8].

Some authors also demonstrated that the significant impact on the quality of life due to psoriasis in children is generally comparable with the effect of other serious pediatric chronic diseases (such as arthritis, diabetes, epilepsy, or asthma).

Skin conditions associated with psoriasis often make the patient more prone to bullying and children could also experience feelings of social stigmatization, especially when skin lesions are localized in visible areas (such as face, scalp, hands) [6–9].

Pediatric patients also had higher risk of being diagnosed with psychiatric comorbidities (such as depression, anxiety, or any other psychiatric disorders) compared with psoriasis-free control subjects [9].

Considering the multidimensional impact of childhood psoriasis, the quality of life in children and adolescents with psoriasis should be strictly monitored, evaluating physical, emotional, and social functioning.

The impact of childhood psoriasis is related not only to the clinical severity of disease, but also to the management and treatment, which generally greatly influence the quality of life of children with psoriasis [10–13].

In fact, the identification of an optimal disease's treatment could be a long and challenging process with several therapeutic attempts.

© The Author(s), under exclusive license to Springer Nature
Switzerland AG 2022
A. Belloni Fortina, F. Caroppo, *Pediatric Psoriasis*,
https://doi.org/10.1007/978-3-030-90712-9_9

Topical therapies can be heavy, demanding, and time-consuming; on the other hand, systemic treatments are often associated with worries and anxiety by parents and family of children, especially in case of prolonged treatments with possible related side-effects [11–13].

The evaluation of the impact on quality of life of psoriasis in children should be an integral part in the management of the disease.

Several tools have been developed to assess the several aspects of quality of life in children with psoriasis.

9.1   Children's Dermatology Life Quality Index (CDLQI)

A simple tool that is commonly used to assess the quality of life related to chronic skin dermatoses in children is the Children's Dermatology Life Quality Index (CDLQI) score.

CDLQI score is calculated through a questionnaire, specifically structured to investigate the quality of life in pediatric age [14, 15].

The questionnaire consists of 10 multiple choice questions with a unique possible answer, exploring several areas of children's life (such as symptoms due to disease, personal sensations, school and sport activities, interpersonal and familiar relationships, and quality of sleep).

The severity of the impact of psoriasis on children's quality of life is classified into five categories based on CLDQI score: no impact on quality of life (CDLQI score: 0–1), small impact on quality of life (CDLQI score: 2–6), moderate impact on quality of life (CDLQI score: 7–12), very large impact on quality of life (CDLQI score: 13–18), extremely large impact on quality of life (CDLQI score: 19–30) [16].

In younger children, a cartoon version of the CDLQI questionnaire has been developed and validated and is commonly used in clinical practice [17].

Several studies reported that the impairment of quality of life in children is related to the clinical severity of disease evaluated with Psoriasis Area Severity Index (PASI) and/or Body Surface Area (BSA) score [10–12].

Furthermore, the impact on quality of life in children with psoriasis seems also related to the presence of skin lesions in visible areas (such as face, hands), underlying the psychological impact of chronic skin diseases, especially in children and adolescents [10–12].

Therefore, the evaluation of severity of pediatric psoriasis should be multidimensional, also considering the tools developed to assess the impact on the quality of life, which could be influenced even with minimal involved body surface area.

9.2   Family Dermatology Life Quality Index (FDLQI)

As many inflammatory chronic skin diseases, psoriasis is known to have a great impact on the lives, not only of the patients, but also of their families.

Family Dermatology Life Quality Index (FDLQI) is a validate dermatology-specific instrument useful to evaluate and quantify the impact on the quality of life of family member of patients with skin diseases [18, 19].

Family members play a central role in the care of patients, especially in children with inflammatory chronic skin diseases; family impact data are potentially important components of the measurement of the overall burden of skin disease which should be evaluated and considered.

FDLQI is a simple and user-friendly tool useful for clinical use, consisting of a questionnaire with 10 multiple choice questions addressed to family members of the patient, with a unique possible answer and with a total score ranging from 0 to 30 [18, 19].

The questionnaire evaluates the impact of skin diseases in family members of the patient, investigating several different aspects of his quality of life (such as emotional, social, physical activities).

The impact of pediatric psoriasis on the quality of life in family members of patients can be very important with a great emotional burden and several negative effects on well-being of family members [19–21].

In clinical evaluation of children with psoriasis, the quality of life of parents and care-givers should be ordinarily evaluated and monitored, considering the possibility of a psychological support.

An improvement of quality of life of family members could help to reduce their emotional burden and could help to establish a supportive relationship with parents which can in turn lead to improved patient compliance and outcomes.

References

1. Eichenfield LF, Paller AS, Tom WL, et al. Pediatric psoriasis: evolving perspectives. Pediatr Dermatol. 2018;35(2):170–81.
2. Ganemo A, Wahlgren CF, Svensson A. Quality of life and clinical features in Swedish children with psoriasis. Pediatr Dermatol. 2011;28:375–9.
3. Krueger GG, Feldman SR, Camisa C, et al. Two considerations for patients with psoriasis and their clinicians: what defines mild, moderate, and severe psoriasis? What constitutes a clinically significant improvement when treating psoriasis? J Am Acad Dermatol. 2000;43:281–5.
4. de Jager ME, van de Kerkhof PC, de Jong EM, et al. A cross-sectional study using the Children's dermatology life quality index (DLQI) in childhood psoriasis: negative effect on quality of life and moderate correlation of DLQI with severity scores. Br J Dermatol. 2010;163:1099–101.
5. Beattie PE, Lewis-Jones MS. A comparative study of impairment of quality of life in children with skin diseases and children with other chronic child diseases. Br J Dermatol. 2006;155:145–51.
6. Mercan S, Kivanc AI. Psychodermatology: a collaboration between psychiatry and dermatology. Turk Psikiyatri Derg. 2006;17(4):305–13.
7. de Jager ME, De Jong EM, Evers AW, et al. The burden of childhood psoriasis. Pediatr Dermatol. 2011;28(6):736–7.
8. Beattie PE, Lewis-Jones MS. A comparative study of impairment of quality of life in children with skin disease and children with other chronic childhood diseases. Br J Dermatol. 2006;155(1):145–51.

9. Kimball AB, Wu EQ, Guerin A, et al. Risks of developing psychiatric disorders in pediatric patients with psoriasis. J Am Acad Dermatol. 2012;67(4):651–657e1–2.
10. Na CH, Chung J, Simpson EL. Quality of life and disease impact of atopic dermatitis and psoriasis on children and their families. Children (Basel). 2019;6(12):133.
11. Caroppo F, Zacchino M, Milazzo E, et al. Quality of life in children with psoriasis: results from a monocentric study. G Ital Dermatol Venereol. 2019 Dec;3
12. Randa H, Todberg T, Skov L, Larsen LS, Zachariae R. Healthrelated quality of life in children and adolescents with psoriasis: a systematic review and meta-analysis. Acta Derm Venereol. 2017;97(5):555–63.
13. Bronckers IM, Paller AS, van Geel MJ, van de Kerkhof PC, Seyger MM. Psoriasis in children and adolescents: diagnosis. Management and comorbidities. Paediatr Drugs. 2015;17(5):373–84.
14. Lewis-Jones MS, Ay F. The Children's dermatology life quality index (CDLQI): initial validation and practical use. Br J Dermatol. 1995;132:942–9.
15. Cardiff University Department of Dermatology and Wound Healing. Children's Dermatology Life Quality Index CDLQI: different language versions. Available at: http://www.dermatology. org.uk/quality/cdlqi/quality-cdlqilanguages.html
16. Waters A, Sandhu D, Beattie P, Ezughah F, Lewis-Jones S. Severity stratification of Children's Dermatology Life Quality Index (CDLQI) scores. Br J Dermatol. 2010;163:121.
17. Holme SA, Man I, Sharpe SL, Dykes PJ, Lewis-Jones MS, Finlay AY. The Children's Dermatology Life Quality Index: validation of the cartoon version. Br J Dermatol. 2003;148:285–90.
18. Basra MKA, Sue-Ho R, Finlay AY. The Family Dermatology Life Quality Index: measuring the secondary impact of skin disease. Br J Dermatol. 2007;156:528–38.
19. Basra MK, Edmunds O, Salek MS, Finlay AY. Measurement of family impact of skin disease: further validation of the Family Dermatology Life Quality Index (FDLQI). J Eur Acad Dermatol Venereol. 2008;22:813–21.
20. Żychowska M, Reich A, Maj J, Jankowska-Konsur A, Szepietowski JC. Impact of childhood psoriasis on Caregivers' quality of life, measured with Family Dermatology Life Quality Index. Acta Derm Venereol. 2020;100(15):adv00244.
21. Kim E, Fischer G. Relationship between PASI and FDLQI in paediatric psoriasis, and treatments used in daily clinical practice. Australas J Dermatol. 2021;62(2):190–4.

Printed in the United States
by Baker & Taylor Publisher Services